SOCCER INJURIES
Their Causes, Prevention and Treatment

Ian Beasley and Bob O'Connor

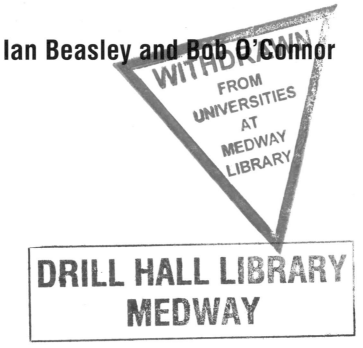
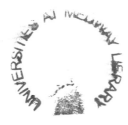

THE CROWOOD PRESS

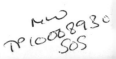

First published in 2006 by
The Crowood Press Ltd
Ramsbury, Marlborough
Wiltshire SN8 2HR

www.crowood.com

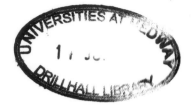

British Library Cataloguing-in-Publication Data
A catalogue record for this book is available from the British Library.

ISBN   1 86126 698 7
EAN   978 1 86126 698 9

Disclaimer

Please note that the authors and the publisher of this book do not
accept any responsibility whatsoever for any error or omission, nor
any loss, injury, damage, adverse outcome or liability suffered as a
result of the information contained in this book, or reliance upon it.
Since soccer and the conditioning and weight training exercises can be
dangerous and could involve activities that are too strenuous for some
individuals to engage in safely, it is essential that a doctor be consulted
before undertaking these activities.

Typeset in Galliard by Bookcraft Ltd, Stroud, Gloucestershire

Printed and bound in Great Britain by Biddles, King's Lynn

Contents

Foreword

With the increasing popularity of our glorious game it is necessary to spread the knowledge of how to prevent and handle injuries, and how to keep players in top condition. Every kind of player, from youth teams to the professionals – men and women, boys and girls – all will profit from this book. While the book is aimed mainly at trainers and doctors, other interested parties such as the players themselves and their parents will find information which is of vital importance to playing the game to the fullest.

Gary Lewin Gard Dip. Phys., MCSP, SRP
Physiotherapist to Arsenal FC and England

Dedication

To my wife Alison, my son Freddie and my daughter Anna whose support allows me to indulge myself in soccer – and who have encouraged me in writing this book.

Ian Beasley

To my son-in-law James Wells, a former soccer player, and my grandson Tyler, who is a budding soccer star.

Bob O'Connor

Introduction

We all know that physical fitness is an essential part of a healthy life. For adults adequate exercise not only makes us feel good it also makes us look better, while keeping our weight and the risks of many diseases under control. Our risk of heart attack, some cancers, diabetes and even the common cold can be greatly reduced. The same benefits apply to young people and in their case participation in sport also allows them to learn to compete and to cooperate as they learn some of the skills necessary for adulthood.

As good as exercise is for us there are occasional downsides to our activities. We may sprain an ankle, suffer a bruise, develop a blister or even break a bone. We now know that exercise can even create some negative by-products in our bodies, such as free oxygen radicals, which we must neutralize if we are to live longer and better.

Effective exercise lowers our depression levels and makes us feel more positive about living. It also reduces the stresses that come from other areas of our lives. Soccer is a team sport, and the ethos of playing on a team can be of help off the field of play, as well as on it.

Soccer is a field sport in which, physiologically, athletes require an aerobic base (that is, they need to be able to keep moving without getting out of breath), and the ability to sprint and recover. There are different amounts of each of these capabilities required for the different positions of play. For instance, central defenders are less physiologically challenged in a game than are midfield players. If a trainer were to ask a defender to play in a midfield role, this player may be physiologically challenged, and rendered more prone to injury. This may be due to the player's inability to maintain position, or to fatigue, or both.

When players start at a soccer club, the trainer may test them for aerobic capacity as well as sprint speed and recoverability. It may be that the player is capable of playing in different positions depending on their physiology, but if not, the trainer needs to know, as a need for substitution may arise in a game where the team needs reorganization and it can affect the outcome of a game.

The medical team may screen or profile the player to try to work out if there is anything obvious that may put the player at a higher risk of injury than normal. There is a debate raging at present within sport as to whether there is any benefit in this, but where there is undoubted benefit is where medical screening for occult disease, such as cardiac screening, can prevent illness or even death.

There are many reasons why a player becomes susceptible to injury. Lack of fitness, strength, 'game intellect' (an understanding of tactics without which players may put themselves into situations which leave them open to injury), nutritional and hydration factors, can all affect susceptibility to injury. This is in addition to the factors inherent in the game: weather conditions such as rain; pitch conditions, such as being hard at the

5

beginning of the season; equipment factors such as unworn shin guards, mouth guards or ankle braces; and the normal risks associated with contact sport.

This book aims to outline the injuries incurred in soccer, how to prevent them or reduce their incidence, and how to treat them. It is essential to recognize the causes of injuries and how often they are likely to occur if we are going to be serious about preventing them – and many can be prevented.

While the trainers and coaches may be more interested in the early chapters, the later chapters are meant for medical personnel. The recommendations will be based on research findings from around the world. Having a better understanding of the body and the major methods of maintaining health, and understanding how to avoid injury and adequately treat injury, can go a long way towards making the game more enjoyable and good health for players more likely.

PART 1

Injuries and Their Prevention

CHAPTER 1

An Overview of Soccer Injuries

An understanding of the types and causes of injuries is essential before we can pursue their prevention and treatment. A number of factors contribute to injuries, such as:

- lack of strength or endurance
- poor balance, boots or shoes, pitch or field surface
- level of play
- heat
- fatigue
- poor nutrition
- foul play
- poor skills
- ineffective officiating.

A player's age and sex are also variables. In order to make the game safer we must be aware of a number of such factors. It is better to prevent the injury than to have to treat it. Before we look at the exact types of injury and their causes, perhaps we should examine some studies that have evaluated the type and prevalence of injuries at varying levels of play, at different ages, and the difference of injury types between the sexes.

Several agencies are seriously research-ing sports injuries and their prevention. FIFA (Fédération Internationale de Football Association) has done a number of studies, particularly for élite-level players. The Oslo Sports Trauma Research Center at the Nor-wegian School for Sport Sciences, directed by Roald Bahr, are major researchers in the field. Julie Steele and Caroline Finch of Aus-tralia are others, but studies are being done in many other countries as well. The Univer-sity of Leicester has for years had a centre for the study of soccer – and injuries and their prevention is a large part of its work. While injury reporting was originally done prima-rily by counting reported injuries, researchers now look at videos of practices and games to see exactly how the injuries occurred. This provides far more insight into how better to prevent many injuries from happening.

TYPES AND FREQUENCY OF SOCCER INJURIES

Lower extremity injuries account for well over half of all soccer injuries. Bruises (contusions) to the thigh and leg, muscle strains to the front or back of the thigh, and ankle sprains are the most common. Many injuries are the result of overuse. Shin splints, stress fractures and knee pain are examples.

The lower back is also a site of pain, usually caused by muscle or connective tissue overuse. The hips and pelvic area can be injured through kicking, while the neck and head are problem areas because of contact with the ball or with other players.

Goalkeepers have a number of finger injuries because of their contact with hard-kicked balls. Diving may also cause arm or wrist fractures and shoulder and collarbone breaks.

LEVEL OF PLAY AND REPORTED INJURIES

Over the years studies have shown quite different frequencies of injuries, possibly because of the way an injury was categorized. As the reporting of injuries has become more standardized, we see that the frequency of reported injuries to the various body parts is becoming more similar (Walden *et al.*, 2005).

Élite Level

A survey of twenty studies of injury frequency has shown that élite soccer players experience between thirteen and thirty-five injuries per thousand hours of competition and 1.5–7.6 per thousand hours of training. For competition this translates to 0.8–2 injuries per match. The most common types of injury were:

- muscle strains (35–37%)
- ligament sprains (20–21%)
- contusions (16–24%).

The areas most commonly affected were:

- thigh (23–24%)
- ankle (18–19%)
- knee (15–17%)
- foot (6–7%).

Contact with another player was shown to be responsible for 44–74% of the injuries.

FIFA developed a standardized injury reporting system to analyse the incidence, circumstances and characteristics of injury during major international football tournaments. It was used in twelve major tournaments, male and female, from 1998 and 2001. A total of 901 injuries were reported from 334 matches, an incidence of 2.7 injuries per match. Injury sites were:

- ankle 17%
- thigh 16%
- head and neck 15%
- lower leg 15%
- knee 12%.

Approximately one injury per match resulted in a player's absence from training or matches. On average 86% of the injuries arose as a result of contact with another player, and approximately half of all injuries were caused by foul play. The number of injuries per match differed substantially between the tournaments for players of different age, sex and skill level. Women's tournaments had fewer injuries than men's tournaments. The highest number of injuries occurred during the Olympic Games and in the Under 20 World Championship (Junge *et al.*, 2004a).

In studying the World Cup of 2002, FIFA found that the incidence of injuries was about the same as it had been in 1994 and 1998. A total of 171 injuries were reported from the 64 matches, which is equivalent to an incidence of 2.7 injuries per match; approximately 1–2 injuries per match resulted in absence from training or matches. More than a quarter of all injuries were incurred without contact with another player, and 73% were contact injuries. Half of the contact injuries, or 37% of all injuries, were caused by foul play as

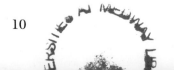

rated by the team physician and the injured player (Junge *et al.*, 2004b). A study of Asian senior and under 20 teams in fifty international tournaments found a higher injury rate than is generally found in the West; however, the patterns of injury were similar.

In a study of 24 male English youth professional players who kept logs of their injuries, it was found that they occurred at only 1.3 injuries per thousand hours of training but 16.3 per thousand hours of game participation. The time off from sport because of the injury averaged twenty days, and of all injuries, 29% were major and 52% were moderate. A poor pitch was involved in 75% of the injuries compared with well-kept fields with 25%. Foul play was the cause of 23.5% of the injuries. Player contact was involved in 48% of the injuries, with tackling the most significant factor. Running, striking and turning accounted for 42% of the injuries. The most common body parts injured were the ankle (28%), foot (13%) and hip (13%). The most common types of injuries were:

- muscle strains (29%)
- ligament sprains (26%)
- contusions or bruises (29%).

The main deficiencies in training methods were in not using shin guards and in not using carbohydrate replacement before and after exercise (Rahnama and Manning, 2004).

Youth Level

A study of injuries in youth soccer in the USA, involving under 12- to under 18-year-old soccer players, over three years (a total of 19,000 player-seasons) with 11,500 players

reporting, showed that girls experienced 0.54 injuries per thousand hours of practice exposures, and 9.81 injuries per thousand hours of game exposures. The rate for boys was 1.06 per thousand hours of practice and 10.89 per thousand hours of playing in matches. For girls 67% of all injuries were to the lower limb including:

- ankle (29%)
- knee (16%)
- lower leg (7%)
- foot (4%)

while 11% of the injuries were to the face.

For boys 65% of the injuries were to the lower limb comprising:

- ankle (22%)
- knee (15%)
- lower leg (9%)
- foot (6%).

Head injuries accounted for 11% of all injuries. The data further indicated that a girls' team might expect 4.01 injuries per season and a boys' team 3.54 injuries per season. About half of those with sprained ankles had had a prior sprain. About 25% of the injuries occurred during the last ten to twelve minutes of a game, probably the result of fatigue. There were also a disproportionate number of injuries early in the season. Both are probably related to fatigue and poor physical condition (Kirkendall *et al.*, 2004).

In a New Zealand study comparing soccer and rugby injuries among boys aged fourteen to eighteen, there were 1.8 injuries per season for the soccer players compared to 2.8 for the rugby players. Two-thirds of all injuries occurred during matches, 20% during training sessions and 15% were overuse injuries (Junge *et al.*, 2004c).

Race and Ethnicity as Possible Factors in Injury

A study of Japanese male youth in the under 12 to under 17 age groups at the National Training Center showed that:

- the under 12 group had 25% of all injuries
- the under 14 group had 30%
- the under 17 group had 44%.

The lower extremity accounted for 73% of all injuries with:

- the under 12 group incurring 67% of all injuries to the lower extremity
- the under 14 group having 86% injuries here
- the under 17 group incurring 64%.

Overuse injuries in the under 12 group accounted for 27% of the injuries, most frequently Osgood–Schlatter disease, the under 14 group had 38% overuse injuries and the under 17 had 35% of their injuries due to overuse (Kohno *et al.*, 2004).

A study of Tunisian professional players showed that there were 4.7 injuries per thousand hours of playing and practising (Junge *et al.*, 2004d). Nearly half of the injuries affected the thigh (hamstrings, quadriceps, abductors and adductors). Most were muscle strains with some muscle tears; 23% of the injuries were ankle sprains with a few knee sprains. This incidence of thigh problems is much higher than is shown in other studies.

Age and Skill

In a one-year study of 398 players aged fourteen to forty-two playing at various levels in the Czech Republic, it was found that the factors related to being injured could be classified as:

- personal: age of player, previous injuries, joint instability, abnormality of the spine, poor physical condition, poor football skills, or inadequate treatment and rehabilitation of injuries
- environmental: exercise overload during practices and games, amount and quality of training, playing field conditions, equipment such as wearing of shin guards and taping, and violations of existing rules or foul play.

During the year they sustained 686 injuries. Of these, 113 (16%) were severe injuries. Ninety-seven severe injuries (86%) were documented in detail. Trauma was the cause of 81% of the injuries and overuse was the cause of 18%. Joint sprains predominated (30%), followed by fractures (16%), muscle strains (15%), ligament ruptures (12%), meniscal tears and contusions (8%), and other injuries. Injuries to the knee were most prevalent (29%), followed by injuries to the ankle (19%) and spine (9%). More injuries occurred during games (59%) than in practice. Of the injured players 24% had suffered a previous injury of the same body part. Contact caused 46% and 54% involved no body contact. Foul play was blamed for 31% of severe injuries (Chomiak *et al.*, 2000).

Gender Factors

In a survey of 202 players during the first two years of the Women's United Soccer Association (WUSA) it was found that a total of 173 injuries occurred to 110 players with an overall injury incidence rate of 1.93 injuries per thousand player hours. The incidence of injury during practice and games was 1.17 and 12.63 per thousand player hours, respectively. Of the injuries 82% were acute and 16% were chronic. Most of the injuries (60%) were located in the lower extremities. Strains (31%), sprains (19%), contusions (16%) and fractures (11%) were the most common diagnoses, and the knee (31%) and head (11%) were the most common sites of injury. Anterior cruciate ligament (ACL) injuries accounted for 5% of all injuries and the incidence of ACL tears was 0.09 per thousand player hours (practice 0.04, game 0.90). Midfielders suffered the most injuries ($p<0.007$). Compared to the male professional league it was concluded that the injury incidence in the WUSA was lower than the 6.2 injuries per thousand player hours found in the corresponding male professional league (Major League Soccer). However, knee injuries predominate even in these élite female athletes (Giza et al., 2005).

In a study of male and female collegiate basketball and soccer players from 1990 to 2002, it was found that females experienced about double the number of anterior cruciate ligament injuries in practice and three times the number in games than did the males. Comparing injury within gender by sport, soccer players consistently sustained more ACL injuries than did basketball players. The rates for all ACL injuries for women were statistically significantly higher than the rates for all ACL injuries for men, regardless of the sport. In soccer, the rate of all ACL injuries across the thirteen years for male soccer players has significantly decreased, whereas it remained constant for female players (Agel et al., 2005).

A Swedish study showed a very high prevalence of knee osteoarthritis, pain and functional limitations in young women who sustained an ACL tear during soccer play twelve years earlier (Lohmander et al., 2004). These findings constitute a strong rationale to direct increased efforts toward prevention and better treatment of knee injuries.

COMMON AREAS OF INJURY

Soft tissue contusions (bruises) are the most common soccer injuries, according to the *American Association of Pediatrics Review*. Fractures are relatively uncommon and account for between 3.5 and 9% of the injuries. In physically immature players, repetitive traction injuries (continual pulling of a muscle on a tendon) are common in the knee and foot. Usually these problems can be helped with a good flexibility programme or activity modification by reducing the amount of running. For heel or foot pain, inserts placed in the soccer shoe may help.

Lower extremity injuries account for up to 81% of all injuries. Of these, 26% are knee injuries and 23% are ankle injuries. However, fractures occur more frequently in the upper extremity than the lower extremity.

Soccer injuries may be traumatic or from overuse. Most (up to 75%) are traumatic. The severity of injuries reported undoubtedly reflects the aggressiveness of the play. More than 75% of players claimed that they were subject to foul play or were badly tackled.

Head Injuries

Head injuries account for between 10% and 13% of all soccer injuries, with concussions accounting for 20% of head injuries.

A Canadian study of players aged ten to twenty-four (Pickett et al., 2005) found that from a total of 1,714 cases of soccer injury identified (an average of 286 a year), 13% were head injuries. The major causative factors for head injury were:

- contact with other players or persons (65%)
- contact with balls (26%).

Heading the ball may not be a major factor in acute injuries to the head but it does not address the possible brain damage from repeated but less forceful heading.

Female athletes sustained a higher percentage of concussions during games than male athletes in a 1997–2000 US study of college athletes. During that time 14,591 injuries incurred in several collegiate sports, and concussions accounted for 6% of all injuries. Females had fewer concussions than males in practice, but in games the females had more concussions. Of all the sports, women's soccer and men's lacrosse were found to have the highest injury rate of concussions. In looking at each sport and combining male and female injuries, it was found that soccer had the greatest number of combined head injuries (Covassin et al., 2003).

More was learned about head injuries in a video study of Norwegian and Icelandic professional games in 1999 and 2000 in which players sustained such injuries. It showed that there were 1.7 such injuries per thousand hours of match play (6% of injuries). Concus-sions occurred at the rate of 0.5 per thousand hours of match play. The most common cause (58%) was a heading duel; 41% of the times it was the opponent's elbow, arm or hand that caused the head injury. The opponent's head was the cause in 32% of the injuries and the foot in 13% of the injuries. Where the arm was involved it was 'active' in 77% of the cases and it was an intentional foul in 20% of the cases (Andersen et al., 2004a).

Spinal Problems

Degenerative change in the spine is seen to begin twenty to thirty years earlier in soccer players than in the general population. Using magnetic resonance imaging (MRI) a study found that older soccer players had more degenerative spinal changes than did younger players and that the soccer players had more and earlier degeneration than the normal population. It was hypothesized that it was because of heading (Kartal et al., 2004).

Neck Injuries

A study of neck injuries in the USA from 1990 to 1999 used data compiled for the US Consumer Product Safety Commission. They were used to generate estimates for the total number of neck injuries and the more specific diagnoses of neck fractures, dislocations, contusions, sprains, strains and lacerations occurring nationally from 1990 to 1999. These data were combined with yearly participation figures to generate rates of injury treated by hospital emergency departments for each sport. Neck injuries were estimated at:

- 5,038 from ice hockey
- 19,341 from soccer
- 114,706 from American football.

The rates for total neck injuries and combined neck contusions, sprains, or strains were higher for American football than for ice hockey or soccer in all years for which data were available. This tells us nothing about the rate of injuries per thousand hours of participation for each sport, though it does indicate that neck injuries are a problem in soccer (Delaney and Al-Kashmiri, 2004).

Ankle Injuries

In a video analysis of Norwegian and Icelandic professional football it was found that there were 46 acute ankle injuries (4.5 per thousand match hours). These were generally player-to-player contacts. The most common were lateral ligament sprains (Andersen, 2004).

In a FIFA study of four world-level competitions there were 76 foot and ankle injuries (52 contusions, 20 sprains, 4 fractures). Direct contact between players was the cause in 72 of them. Significantly more injuries involved a tackle from the side and a lateral or medial tackle force. The injured limb was weight-bearing in 41 and non-weight-bearing in 35 of the incidents. Significantly more injuries resulting in time lost from soccer occurred when the limb was weight-bearing. The most common foot and ankle positions at the time of injury were slightly turned out (pronated) for weight-bearing legs, and slightly turned inward (plantar flexed) for non-weight-bearing legs (Giza et al., 2003).

Other Severe Injuries in Non-Professional Soccer

In a South African study noting only hospital admissions to one hospital, 32 patients were admitted with severe injuries during a 42-month period. The types of injury in this group were similar to soccer injuries reported in other countries. The injuries included eighteen fractures of the tibial and femoral shaft. Two tibial shaft fractures were compound. Four tibial plateau fractures and five epiphyseal injuries were identified. One patient had a fracture-dislocation of the hip. One patient had a popliteal artery injury that developed 48 hours after another injury had occurred, and had an above-knee amputation. In the same period 122 patients were treated as outpatients. The researchers concluded that very serious injuries are sustained by casual soccer players in South Africa and that urgent measures need to be taken to prevent such injuries.

The authors of this study concluded that the fact that 75% of the shaft fractures were related to a direct tackle is disturbing. Uncontrolled aggression on the field and poor football skills appear to be important factors. They therefore concluded that the most important factors contributing to severe injuries in South African community soccer players are their psychological attitudes to the game and towards their opponents, foul play, poor training, and poor physical facilities such as the playing surface (Goga and Gongal, 2003).

CHAPTER 2

Causes of Injuries

In this chapter we will look at how the injuries described in Chapter 1 come about. An understanding of the causes of injury will be critical in addressing the possible preventions that might be considered. These preventative ideas will be addressed in Chapters 4 to 7.

FOUL PLAY

Video recording has advanced research in this field. In Norwegian professional soccer about 40% of all high-risk situations, and about 30% of the injuries identified on video that resulted in free kicks being awarded, were the result of foul play. The conclusion was that there may need to be an improvement in the laws of the game to protect players from unnecessary injury (Andersen *et al.*, 2004b). But a Swedish study found that only about 20% of the injuries were a result of foul play (Walden *et al.*, 2005).

A FIFA study of twelve tournaments used video recordings to analyse 148 general injuries and 84 injuries to the head and neck. The match referees identified 47% of the injuries as caused by fouls, but an expert panel in their video analysis found 69% of the general injuries to have been so caused. For the head and neck injuries the on-field referees ruled that 40% of the injuries had been caused by fouls while the panel found it to be 49%. They concluded that the current rules of football were adequate for the majority of tackle situations, although the reliability with which referees could identify fouls during some match conditions was low (Fuller *et al.*, 2004a).

HEADING

Among college soccer injuries resulting from collisions with fixed objects or other players, around 5% are concussions. These temporary disruptions of the brain's function, caused when the brain is jarred inside its protective skull, trigger symptoms ranging from mild disorientation to unconsciousness. According to the National Collegiate Athletic Association, concussions are about as common in soccer as they are in American football and are more frequent than in other less contact-oriented sports. In the other sports, however, players do not use their heads as they do in soccer. Researchers have not yet determined exactly how much force a headed soccer ball puts on the brain.

Heading – redirecting the ball with the forehead – is essential to the game. In amateur leagues, a player might head the ball six to eight times in a game, and more often during practice. The question is, do all those bumps eventually add up to significant brain injury?

The question of whether heading causes

serious injuries in soccer has long been studied; it is difficult to answer when the heading does not result in an acute injury like a concussion. Repeated lower level traumas, such as occur in boxing, are now being evaluated. In boxing, a person who has never been knocked out may still exhibit reduced brain capacity in one or several areas such as vision, hearing, coordination or memory. Similarly, a soccer player who has never had a concussion may exhibit signs of reduced brain function. When comparing a blow to the head in boxing with one in heading, bear in mind that a punch will generally have more weight behind it than a kicked ball, but the *speed* of the punch and the kicked ball may be quite similar.

Despite the game's popularity and the possibility of head injuries, only a few researchers have looked at the effects of heading in soccer. Several small, preliminary studies now suggest that soccer players are more likely to have problems with memory and planning than are track and field athletes or swimmers. However, these studies have many flaws, their critics point out. Gary Green of the University of California, Los Angeles School of Medicine, for example, maintains that it's difficult to isolate the effects of heading from the effects of other head injuries that soccer players suffer.

Estimates of the number of times a soccer player heads a ball vary from an average of five to nine per game, with European players heading most frequently. One group has uncovered a dose–response relation between headers per season and poor results on cognitive tests. Performance on neuropsychological testing can vary according to the position on the field, with forward and defensive players exhibiting more impairment (Matser *et al.*, 2001).

Erik Matser of The Netherlands studied 53 Dutch male professional soccer players and 27 men who were track and field athletes or swimmers. Soccer players fared slightly worse on tests of memory, planning and visual–spatial relations than the other athletes. Among the soccer players, those who had suffered the most concussions fared worse on those tests than players with fewer head injuries. Furthermore, those who played forward or defensive positions, where people are most likely to head the ball, showed slightly more impairment than those who played midfield. The most striking differences appeared in a test that required people to copy a complex figure and then draw it from memory. Compared with established standards, 7% of the non-soccer athletes and 45% of professional soccer players had moderately to significantly impaired scores (Matser *et al.*, 1998).

Matser contends that while most sports physicians believe that proper heading does not cause brain injury, a direct, full-power blow from a soccer ball kicked by an adult has about the same force as a boxer's punch. Young players encounter less force. They play with smaller balls and cannot kick them as hard as adults can. Moreover, many children under twelve in organized soccer are discouraged from heading in practice and games.

Many years ago Ernst Jokl developed his theory about injuries to the head in boxing. He found that when the head receives a blow, the brain moves violently within the cranium. If there are rough edges where the skull bones connect the brain may experience very small traumas, which he called 'pinpoint haemorrhages'. A small scar then developed. If these microscopic injuries continued, a greater area of microscopic scarring developed. Then, depending on the area of the brain affected, the boxer would gradually lose memory, vision, coordination, hearing or other brain capacities. It might also be noted that a skilled boxer will 'slip' many punches by moving his head away from the punch, but a soccer player in many cases will attempt to absorb the whole force of the ball when redirecting it.

There are two ways heading might cause brain injury, according to Matser. If a person heads a ball properly, attacking it with the top part of the forehead, the force of the blow affects the front and back of the brain. As the head contacts the ball, the brain sloshes forward against the front of the skull, then it rebounds and hits the back of the skull. A more recent theory is that the heavier spinal fluid is forced forward initially, forcing the brain to the rear of the skull. The brain then rebounds and hits the front of the cranium. This may account for the fact that greater injuries are usually observed in the back of the brain than the front from frontal blows to the head.

What is more dangerous than a frontal header, according to Matser, is when a player heads a ball to either side of the forehead, slightly rotating the skull, so that the brain can twist on its stem. Such twisting may cause breaks in the links between nerve cells, a kind of damage known as 'diffuse axonal injury'. 'Experience with boxing suggests that there is no question that repeated blows to the head can cause central nervous system damage', notes David Abwender of the State University of New York at Brockport. 'Heading is a relatively minor impact, but an impact nonetheless. This may put a person at risk for very slight nerve damage that, over time, may lead to impairment' (Abwender, 1999).

There are several scientific means of measuring forces to the head. These are used to ascertain forces in simulated traffic accidents and in sporting head trauma situations, and are utilized in evaluating the safety of sports helmets, such as in skiing, biking and football. The Gadd Severity Index is a commonly used measure. According to its scale, a level of 1,000 would be life threatening. In a study of 38 college football players (Duma *et al.*, 2005) during 45 sessions, over 3,300 impacts were recorded. The average impact experienced averaged 36, with a range of 7 to 57. A mild concussion was the result of an impact on the helmet that measured 267.

In another study using the Gadd Severity Index, forces to the skull experienced in a game of American football and hockey were compared, with measuring devices in the helmets. American football averaged 29.2G (gravity force) compared with 35G for hockey. The researchers then went to the laboratory to measure the impact of heading a soccer ball while wearing an American football helmet. The result was an average impact of 54.7G, nearly 90% greater than the average blow to an American football player while tackling (Naunheim *et al.*, 2000). That figure would probably have been much higher if the soccer players had not used football helmets.

Possible Effects of Heading

How do soccer players compare with other athletes when it comes to brain injury? In another study by the Dutch researcher Matser, adult amateur soccer players fared worse on tests of planning and memory than did swimmers or track and field athletes. The number of concussions an individual had suffered was inversely related to performance on six of the sixteen tests. Roughly similar percentages of athletes in the two groups suffered concussions unrelated to soccer. Almost half of the soccer players had suffered at least one soccer-related concussion, however.

> Although [soccer-related] cognitive impairment appears to be mild, it presents a medical and public health concern since there are 200 million registered amateur and professional soccer players worldwide...Our results indicate that participation in amateur soccer, in general, and concussion, specifically, is associated with impaired performance in memory and planning functions. Due to the worldwide popularity of soccer, these observations may have important public health implications.
>
> Matser *et al.* (1999)

Another small study reported at a meeting of the American Psychological Association in Boston suggests that a lifetime of soccer playing might lead to mental deficits substantial enough to cause problems with a person's social life or ability to perform his or her job. Compared with a similar group of swimmers, twenty-six college-age men and women who had played soccer scored similarly on eleven mental tests (Abwender, 1999). However, a group of six professional soccer players consistently fared worse on these tests than older swimmers and college-age soccer players and swimmers. Despite these results, the link between heading and brain damage is still often seen as controversial.

Further evidence comes from a Swedish study (Stalnacke *et al.*, 2004), which measured in male soccer players two biochemical markers that indicate brain tissue damage. Blood samples were taken from players before and after a competitive game and the numbers of headers and of trauma events during soccer play were assessed. Both markers were significantly raised in samples obtained after the game. One was nearly doubled. The increases were significantly related to the number of headers performed in a match.

Possible, But Not Proven, Effects of Heading

Trauma has long been hypothesized, but never proven, to be a risk factor for amyotrophic lateral sclerosis (ALS), sometimes called Lou Gehrig's disease. This hypothesis may now have a renaissance due to recent reports in the lay press on the 'Italian motoneuron mystery', that is, the disclosure of thirty-three diagnosed ALS cases in a subpopulation of 24,000 soccer players of the top three Italian divisions from the 1960s to 1996. Thirteen have already died of the disease. This is a rate of 132 per hundred thousand. (The global rate is 0.6 to 2.6 per hundred thousand.) Could the repetitive brain trauma of heading represent an environmental risk factor for developing ALS in genetically predisposed individuals? Additionally the normal age at onset of ALS is 63.8 years but in Italian soccer players the onset averaged in the 40–50 age range. A review of the literature (*see* Piazza *et al.*, 2004) offers some interesting perspectives.

Since strenuous exercise could be considered to be a possible cause of ALS, Italian cyclists were evaluated. Of the six thousand cyclists who had competed during the last thirty years none had developed ALS. If exercise were the cause of the disease in soccer players we might have expected to have eight cases among the cyclists.

ALS may be related to a combination of genetic susceptibility and environmental factors, such as:

- a history of trauma to the brain and spinal cord
- strenuous physical activity
- exposure to lead, radiation, electrical shocks, welding or soldering materials
- employment in paint, petroleum or dairy industries.

So while there is no known connection between heading a soccer ball and developing ALS, there are indications that repeated head trauma may be a factor as in other brain problems.

Compared to individuals with other neurological diseases, patients with ALS are more likely to have a history of being athletic and slim, according to Scarmeas *et al.* (2002).

Hints of such a connection have been floating around for years. Boxer Ezzard Charles, baseball player Catfish Hunter and, of course, baseball icon Lou Gehrig all died of ALS. Three players from the San Francisco Fortyniners football team were diagnosed with ALS in the 1980s, and Glenn Montgomery of the Seattle Seahawks lost his life to ALS in 1998. All were athletic and slim. Is ALS only caused by genes or may genes predispose some people depending on their environmental experiences?

There have been reports linking head trauma to Parkinson's disease (Mohammed Ali may be a case in point), Alzheimer's disease and schizophrenia. No links are yet proven, only hypothesized.

While a soccer ball weighs only 400–450g, it can be kicked at a speed in excess of 75 miles an hour (120km/h). Soccer kicks, when headed, are commonly estimated to generate 500–1200 newtons to the forehead. This is sufficient force to fracture a cheekbone. (A newton is one kilogram per metre per second.) A boxer's hard punch to the head would be near 6,300 newtons, assuming that the boxer did not slip the punch.

Head trauma is a known risk factor for adult dementia in the presence of a predisposing genetic condition (Guo *et al.*, 2000). It has also been reported in retired professional footballers (Barnett and Curran, 2003). A relationship between soccer and dementia is still a matter of speculation. A smaller study (Sortland and Tysvaer, 1989) found that onethird of the players studied had central cerebral atrophy, probably caused by repeated small head injuries in connection with heading the ball. A coroner's court ruled that professional soccer player Jeff Astle's death was related to his regularly heading the ball, a skill for which he was famous (Eaton, 2002).

There May Be No Problem in Heading

Several of the above-cited studies failed to examine the subjects' concussion history, so measures of mental impairment may have more to do with a prior history of concussions – either on or off the soccer field – than with heading, according to Jim Moorhouse of the US Soccer Federation in Chicago. He maintains that it is far from clear that deficits in performance on the sensitive neurologic tests that researchers use translate into real-life problems. No study has yet shown that soccer players are more likely than other athletes to have trouble with relationships, difficulty remembering things, or problems performing their jobs.

Jordan Metzl of the Hospital for Special Surgery in New York agrees. 'What works in a lab doesn't always hold true in real life,' he argues. 'I think the risk [of mental impairment] from concussion is real, but I'm not convinced by the available information on repetitive heading,' he says. However, Abwender (1999) argues, 'data are starting to paint a coherent picture that playing soccer for many years can present a risk' of mental impairment.

The views are somewhat different regarding children who play soccer. 'There is as yet no compelling evidence to suggest that, in the absence of frank concussion, younger soccer athletes are at particular risk for [mental] impairment,' said Abwender. He is not yet convinced that heading should be banned even from youth soccer. Some researchers disagree. Simple common sense suggests that headers should be banned among younger players, according to Frank Webbe of the Florida Institute of Technology in Melbourne.

In the mid-1990s, observation of the US national team and of Swedish soccer players failed to link repeated heading with any mental impairment. Broglio et al.'s 2004 study involved college soccer players who headed twenty balls hurled at a speed of 55 miles per hour (88.71km/h), and were then tested for body sway as an indication of coordination. The results indicated that there was no real difference between the coordination of those who headed the balls and those who did not.

While heading the ball may be a factor in brain injury, other factors related to the heading attempt may be more important, especially for the more harmful injuries. Head-to-head contact is probably a greater danger in terms of the single contact, and the use of arms above the head while attempting to head the ball may also be a factor in more serious injury. Of course this does not address the possibility of cumulative brain injuries by heading the ball in practice or in games.

TACKLING

It is fairly clear what kinds of tackle cause injury. Another FIFA study (Fuller et al., 2004b) analysed tackling injuries in 123 matches in FIFA tournaments and found that tackles from the side were twice as likely to require post-match medical attention as tackles from behind. Injuries to the head and/or neck of tackled and tackling players and the torso of tackling players were the most serious. Injuries to the foot for tackled and tackling players and the lower leg and thigh for tackling players were less serious. Tackles with risk to the tackled players involved the crashing of heads and two-footed tackles. For those doing the tackling risks were from the clashing of heads, two-footed tackles, jumping vertically, and tackles from the side. It was concluded that the laws of football relating to tackling should be reviewed to provide greater protection from injury by reducing the overall level of risk and, in particular, by protecting players from high-risk tackles.

Tackling and Player Error

Tackling was evaluated using 123 videos of FIFA international matches (Fuller et al., 2004c). A total of 8,572 tackles were assessed, of which 40% were fouls. There were 299 incidents of on-pitch medical attention, of which 44% resulted from foul tackles, and 200 post-match team physicians' reports, of which 48% resulted from foul tackles. Tackled players received 74% of the post-match medical reports. Tackle types with the greatest probability of requiring medical attention were from the side in terms of tackle direction, jumping vertically in terms of tackle mode, and a clash of heads in terms of tackle action. Human error in terms of illegal tackling on the part of players during the process of tackling and inadequacies in the laws of football and/or their application by match referees were equally responsible for the high levels of injury observed.

PREVIOUS INJURY

This appears to be a significant factor in injury, and featured highly in a study of factors relative to injuries in the two highest divisions in Icelandic soccer (Arnason *et al.*, 2004). At the beginning of the season 306 players were evaluated for height, weight, body composition, flexibility, leg extension power, jump height, peak O_2 uptake, joint stability, and history of previous injury. Charting all the injuries, it was found that the older players had about 10% more injuries than the younger players. They were about 40% more likely to suffer a hamstring injury than the younger players. But *any* player with a previous hamstring strain was eleven times more likely to incur one again. A previous groin injury increased the chances of incurring another by seven times. Previous injury was also found to increase knee injuries by four times and ankle sprains by five times.

SUMMARY OF INJURIES

While the previously cited studies include various populations – male and female; European, American, Asian and African; youth to élite; and young to old – there are some similarities and concerns. To summarize, of all injuries:

- 65–80% involved the lower extremity
- 6–14% were head injuries
- 13–23% were ankle injuries
- 15–30% were muscle strains
- 12–32% were ligament sprains.

As to the causes of injury:

- foul play was identified in 31–69% of the reported injuries
- contact with another player accounted for 70–80% of the injuries
- older players and players with previous injuries had more injuries than younger or uninjured players
- overuse injuries ranged from 17% to 35% of the total injuries
- females had two to three times the number of knee injuries, especially ACL injuries.

These factors should be addressed to make the game safer for the millions who play it.

CHAPTER 3

The Athletic Body

In Chapter 1 we looked at the incidence of soccer injuries. Before we examine preventative strategies and treatment possibilities we must understand the makeup of the tissues that can be injured when playing. Although anatomy is not always the most accessible subject, it is important to have a general grasp of how the brain, muscles, tendons and ligaments work in order to have a better understanding of how to prevent and treat injuries and how more effectively to train athletes for better performance.

THE BRAIN

The initiation of any movement, be it running, kicking, or jumping, occurs in the brain. Input from the eyes, and interpretations in the brain (game intellect), causes the motor cortex in the brain to send electro-chemical messages to the appropriate muscles to make the body move in the desired way.

There are billions of neurons that make up the brain. Messages are sent from one part of the brain to another or to the muscles through electro-chemical circuits. Electricity passes down the nerve, and when it reaches the end, chemical neurotransmitters are released that move to the end of the next nerve and stimulate it to start another electric current which will run the length of that nerve. This sequence of electrical to chemical to electrical to chemical may happen thousands of times between the part of the brain where an idea is produced to a muscle. When the signal arrives, the muscle contracts and elicits a shortening of the muscle, resulting in movement.

There are hundreds of different neurotransmitters in the brain and lower body. When the nerve is damaged, as it may be from blows to the head or from alcohol, it fails to conduct the electricity. On the other hand, the neurotransmitters can be increased or decreased from naturally occurring phenomena, such as arousal for a soccer game or clinical depression. They can also be influenced by other things, such as food. For example milk, which is high in the amino acid tryptophan, may increase the neurotransmitter serotonin, which helps us to relax and sleep. Coffee, on the other hand, may increase noradrenaline and make us more alert. Psychoactive drugs, both legal and illegal, affect the neurotransmitters by increasing or decreasing them in various parts of the brain. Such drugs as marijuana, cocaine, ecstasy, methamphetamines and heroin affect mood because of their effects on the neurotransmitters.

The brain rests in the cranium of the skull and is cushioned by cerebrospinal fluid. Injuries can occur to the brain when a blow deadens an area of the brain (concussion) or when small areas of the brain are damaged by pinpoint haemorrhages from small injuries. Of course there can also be genetic, bacterial and viral causes to health problems in the brain.

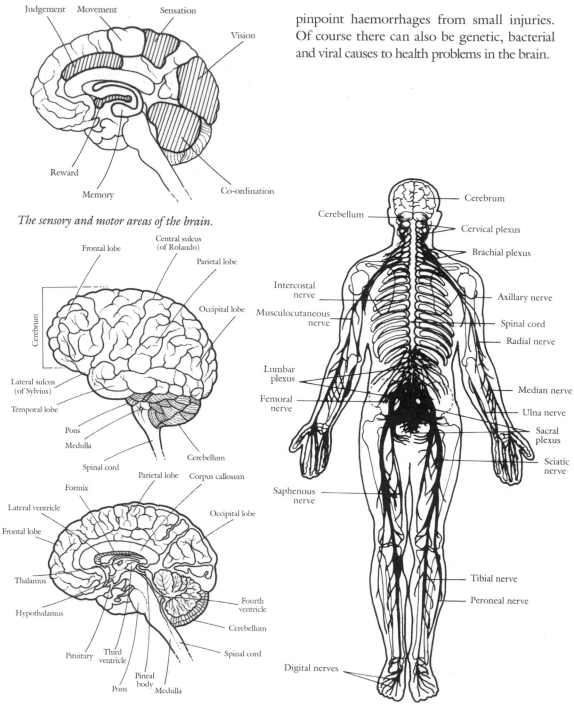

The sensory and motor areas of the brain.

Exterior and interior of the brain.

The nervous system.

BONES: THE SKELETAL SYSTEM

The muscular system that allows us to move does so by using bones as levers. Bones are unusual in that the bone itself is one organ, and it encloses another organ, the bone marrow. The marrow's function is to produce the various types of blood cells, both white and red.

Bones are thought of as being solid organs that do not change that much. However, like the rest of the body, there is a turnover throughout life in bone that causes it to be remodelled in response to the stresses it is put under.

For instance, the bone density in the dominant arm in professional tennis players is greater than in the non-dominant arm. It is also known that weight-bearing exercise is a highly effective method of building stronger bones all through life and even in women after the menopause. The bone strengthens itself in response to the stress of weight-bearing exercise. Bed rest, on the other hand, will allow the bones to decompose and weaken.

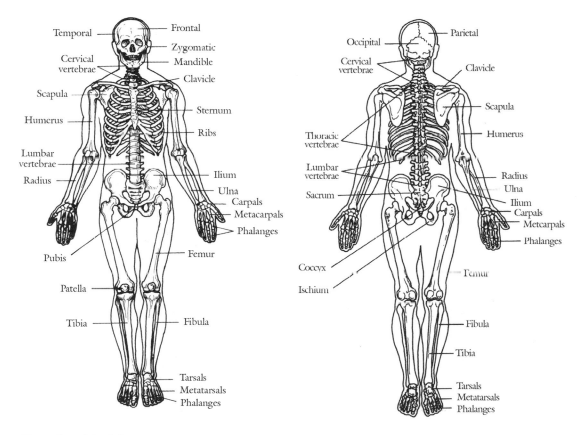

Front view of the skeleton.

Back view of the skeleton.

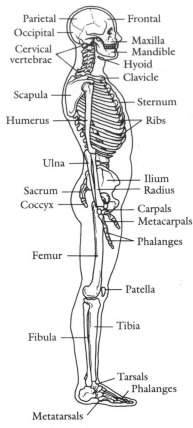

Side view of the skeleton.

Labels on skeleton diagram: Parietal, Occipital, Cervical vertebrae, Scapula, Humerus, Ulna, Sacrum, Coccyx, Femur, Fibula, Metatarsals, Frontal, Maxilla, Mandible, Hyoid, Clavicle, Sternum, Ribs, Ilium, Radius, Carpals, Metacarpals, Phalanges, Patella, Tibia, Tarsals, Phalanges

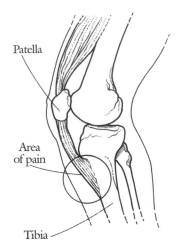

Osgood–Schlatter disease.

Labels: Patella, Area of pain, Tibia

Before adulthood, there are areas of bone that are called growth plates. These are made up of soft immature bone cells, which lay down new bone cells in layer upon layer, not unlike sedimentation on a seabed, thereby making the bone bigger or longer. In long bones, these are near the end, but can be at differing sites in other bones. As might be expected, if severely injured, and the growth plate is disturbed, the normal pattern of growth and maturity can be altered, causing biomechanical problems later on. For instance if the growth plate of the upper tibia (shinbone) is injured, growth can be interrupted, resulting in a difference in leg length. A common com-

plaint in young footballers is Osgood–Schlatter disease. It is the result of repeated pulling on the growth plate of the upper tibia by the quadriceps tendon when running. The quadriceps tendon attaches just below the knee-cap so whenever the knee is straightened, such as when running or jumping, the bone plates at the top of the tibia are pulled outward. This results in pain when playing, but usually has no long-term implications. It does, however, show us how the growth plate can respond to trauma, and why we should always be careful when exercising children too excessively.

CONNECTIVE TISSUE

There are a number of connective tissues that hold other tissues together. There is tissue that holds one microscopic muscle cell to another, and there are ligaments that connect one bone to another. Tendons attach muscles to bone.

Connective tissue tends to shorten as we age. This is one of the reasons for doing lifelong flexibility exercises. Connective tissues, like bones, are active tissues. Strength training will increase the size and strength of the tendons. Vitamin C will help to form the collagen that is one of the ingredients in the connective tissues.

Ligaments

Joints are formed of bones and ligaments. The ligaments are tight enough to hold the bones together but placed in such a way that the bones can move through their appropriate joint action. In the knee, for instance, the collateral ligaments are on the inside and the outside of the joint, just below the skin, and help prevent the joint from moving in a 'knock-kneed' or 'bow-legged' way. The knee joint is special as it has two large ligaments inside the joint itself, called the cruciate ligaments (so called because they cross over each other, as in a crucifix). There is one that arises at the front (anterior cruciate ligament, or ACL), and one at the back (posterior, or PCL). These ligaments help stop the knee sliding across itself forwards or backwards, and help prevent rotational injuries. The ligaments in the knee prevent it from hyper-extending – the lower leg moving past the vertical with the ankle forward of the knee.

Of course, in sport, any ligament can be injured, sometimes requiring surgery. A stretched ligament is called a sprain. A blow to the outside of the knee might bend the knee inward and stretch the ligament on the inside of the knee (the medial collateral ligament). A blow from the inside of the knee may bend it outward and stretch the ligament on the outside of the knee – the lateral collateral ligament. The anterior cruciate ligament is probably the most commonly injured of the knee ligaments.

Ankle ligaments, particularly those on the outside of the ankle, are commonly sprained. In the spine ligaments hold the vertebrae close to each other. They can be stretched in road traffic accidents in which the neck is 'whiplashed' or by a blow to the head by a soccer ball or an opponent.

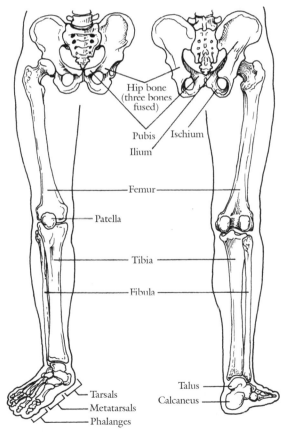

Hip bone
(three bones fused)

Pubis   Ischium

Ilium

Femur

Patella

Tibia

Fibula

Talus
Calcaneus

Tarsals
Metatarsals
Phalanges

The hip and leg from the front and rear.

Tendons

Tendons connect muscle to bone. They, like ligaments, are made of very strong fibrous tissue. They can transmit great forces in movement when a powerful muscle contraction moves a bone quickly. The biceps tendon can be felt just inside the elbow. Compare the large quadriceps muscle at the front of the thigh, and the small width of the quadriceps tendon that is easily felt at the front of the knee, when the joint is bent to 90 degrees. Some tendons (e.g. those around the ankle and wrist), travel in sheaths of synovium (see below), so that smooth movements may be achieved. Surrounding the synovium is a tunnel of generic connective tissue, giving protection to the whole mechanism. These sheaths can themselves be injured and cause pain or discomfort, and interrupt the smooth movements that may be required, in absolute contradiction of their purpose. Tendons can be ruptured or strained.

This connective tissue membrane condenses at each end of the muscle. At one end of the muscle there is an attachment to bone that acts as an 'anchor'. This is usually at the end closest to the centre of the body (the proximal end). The other end of the muscle narrows down, and forms a tendon, which is attached to the bone as well, but this attachment is the other side of a joint (the distal end).

When the muscle contracts concentrically (as opposed to eccentrically; *see* Glossary), it shortens, and pulls on the tendon, which then moves the joint concerned. A good example of this is the quadriceps (the muscle at the front of the thigh). The anchors for the various parts of this muscle are in the pelvis. The tendon attachment is found just below the front of the knee joint. When the muscle is contracted, the knee straightens. On the contrary, the hamstring muscle, at the back of thigh, has its origins in the pelvis also, and its contraction also pulls on a tendon below the knee,

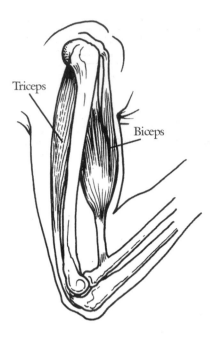

The biceps and triceps tendons.

but in the rear. The action of the hamstrings causes the knee to bend (flex). The actions of the quadriceps and hamstrings oppose each other, and are described as 'antagonistic' to each other.

MUSCLES

The smallest functional unit of a muscle is called a sarcomere. The sarcomere is made up of two proteins, myosin and actin. When the brain signals the muscle to contract, the actin proteins slide towards each other on the myosin. They are pulled by what we call crossbridges. While we do not know what a crossbridge looks like we assume that there

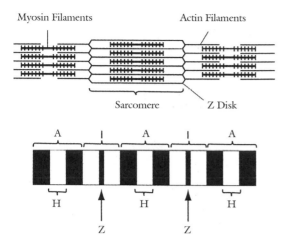

Myosin Filaments   Actin Filaments

Sarcomere   Z Disk

A sarcomere. Source: O'Connor, 2001

sarcomere, such as in the hamstrings while running, when the body is programmed to relax the muscles on one side of the joint when the muscles on the other side of the joint are contracting. This is called reciprocal innervation. The sarcomeres can also lengthen when under tension, such as when a heavy weight is held in the hand as at the end of a biceps curl, then the weight slowly lowered.

The other type of sarcomere action is an isometric contraction (isometric means 'same length'). Here the muscle tightens but doesn't shorten. This type of action would frequently occur in the neck when heading the ball.

Most muscle strains seem to occur during the eccentric action. As the muscle is stretched, the actin may be torn from the myosin, being stretched away so that no crossbridges attach the two protein elements of the sarcomere.

The potential power of a sarcomere depends on it having both the room to contract, to move the actin a sufficient distance on the myosin, and to have enough crossbridges connecting the actin and the myosin so that enough force can be generated. There are several states that a sarcomere may have.

must be some element that allows the actin to crawl up on the myosin.

Sarcomeres in Action

There are three actions that a sarcomere can make. It can contract or shorten (a concentric action). This happens in the muscles in the front of the thigh (quadriceps) when the thigh is brought forward in running. At the same time there is a stretching action in the muscles in the back of the thigh (hamstrings and gluteals). The sarcomeres in the hamstrings are lengthening in what is called an eccentric action. 'Eccentric' means 'unusual'. So a sarcomere, which has the usual action of shortening, is lengthening as a result of a force. While it is sometimes called an eccentric *contraction* that would be impossible because to contract means to shorten and in an eccentric action the muscle is lengthening. The lengthening action can be without tension in the

- A contracture occurs when the actin has moved nearly all the way up the myosin. There are many crossbridges connecting the actin and myosin but there is little or no room for additional contraction to take place. This is abnormal and may have to be corrected by surgery or by putting the limb in a cast and stretching it. Muscular dystrophy is an example of a disease with serious contractures.
- A stiff muscle (sarcomere) has some room for contraction, because there are a number of crossbridges connecting the actin and myosin. A stiff muscle is helpful

in running, even distance running, because the stiffness factor acts to increase running efficiency even without the contraction of the sarcomere – probably acting somewhat like a rubber band, stretching then returning to the original position.

- A normal state in which the actin has sufficient crossbridges to grip the myosin effectively and enough room to make a meaningful contraction.

- An over-compliant sarcomere would have a long gap in which to move the actin over the myocin but relatively few crossbridges connecting the two to generate much force. This may happen when the sarcomere has been overstretched in passive static stretching.

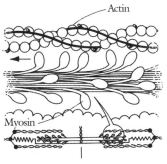

Relaxed

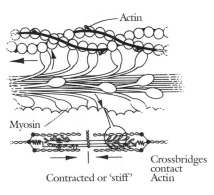

Contracted or 'stiff'

Actin–myosin relationships.

- A torn or strained sarcomere in which there are few or no crossbridges connecting the actin and myocin and damage has occurred.

The drawing on the left is a simplified illustration of what stiffness or lack of stiffness in a muscle may imply. Other factors that influence stiffness are:

- the whole muscle–tendon complex
- the amount of neural stimulation
- other elements within the sarcomere (i.e. titin), and
- some properties in the sarcomere that increase stiffness independent of the number of crossbridges activated.

The sarcomeres are connected end to end in a muscle thread (myofibril). It is estimated that there are 4,000 to 10,000 sarcomeres per myofibril laid end to end. Each is about one ten-thousandth of a centimetre long. There are five to ten thousand myofibrils in a muscle fibre and about 250,000 fibres in the biceps muscle. So we are talking about a lot of sarcomeres.

The sarcomeres and fibres are not identical. There are what are called fast and slow twitch muscle fibres. Fast twitch or type IIB fibres contract five to twenty-five times faster than the slow twitch or type I fibres. But the slow twitch fibres can continue to contract for relatively long periods. Then there are intermediate fibres, or type IIA, which can adapt in either direction, fast or slow, depending on how they are trained. There are actually even more fibre types but the three mentioned are by far the most prevalent. These muscle proteins are 'hung' in a connective tissue skeleton, and appear as

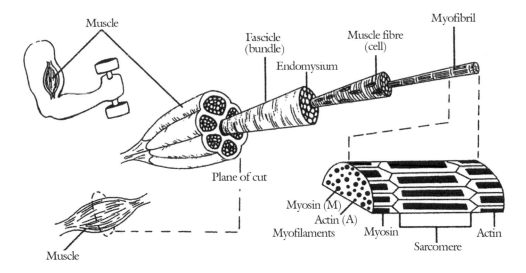

Structure of muscle fibres. Source: O'Connor, 2001

the fine membranes that can be seen within red meat.

When a muscle strain occurs, as it does quite frequently in the hamstrings during a soccer match, the sarcomeres or myofibrils can be stretched and broken. In major strains a large number of these fibres can be overstretched or destroyed.

A Closer Look at Muscle Architecture

A single muscle fibre is a cyclindrical, elongated cell. Muscle cells can be extremely short, or long. The sartorious muscle contains single fibres that are at least 30cm long. Each fibre is surrounded by a thin layer of connective tissue called endomysium.

Organizationally, thousands of muscle fibres are wrapped by a thin layer of connective tissue called the perimysium to form a muscle bundle. Groups of muscle bundles that join into a tendon at each end are called muscle groups, or simply muscles. The biceps

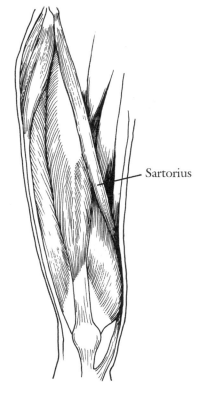

Sartorius muscle with quadriceps.

31

muscle is an example. The entire muscle is surrounded by a protective sheath called the epimysium. Between and within the muscle cells is a complex latticework of connective tissue, resembling struts and crossbeams, that helps to maintain the integrity of the muscle during contraction and strain. It is an amazing cellular system, even before it starts working.

Interior components of the muscle cell

Every muscle cell contains a series of common components that are directly associated with muscle contraction in some way, and that are influenced by training.

- *Cell membrane* This controls what enters and leaves the cell. It contains regulatory proteins that are influenced by hormones like adrenalin (epinephrine) and insulin. The blood concentration of these hormones greatly influences fuel utilization by the muscle cell.
- *Contractile proteins* The contractile machinery of a muscle fibre, as previously mentioned, is organized into structural units called sarcomeres. Muscle length is determined by how many sarcomeres are lined up in series, connected end to end. Muscle thickness ultimately depends on how many sarcomeres line up in parallel (one on top of the other).
- *Cytosol* This is the aqueous fluid of the cell. It provides a medium for diffusion and movement of oxygen, new proteins and ATP (adenosine triphosphate) within the cell. The cytoplasm also contains glycogen (sugar), lipid (fat) droplets, phosphocreatine, various chemical ions like magnesium, potassium and chloride, and numerous enzymes.

- *Mitochondria* These are the organelles in each muscle cell that contain oxidative enzymes which consume oxygen during exercise. Recent research suggests that mitochondria may look more like an interconnected network than the little isolated oval 'powerhouses' shown in most old textbooks. Mitochondria convert the chemical energy contained in fat and carbohydrate to ATP (adenosine tri-phosphate), the only energy source that can be used directly by the cell to cause a muscle contraction. Ultimately, glucose and fat molecules (and certain amino acids) break down and combine with oxygen to form ATP, carbon dioxide, water and heat energy. This occurs via enzymatic processes occurring first in the cytosol and then the mitochondria. The carbon dioxide and excess water leave the body through our breath. The ATP generated provides a usable energy source for muscle contraction and other cell functions. Heat removal occurs by sweating and as radiant heat transfer from the skin to the surrounding air. Clearly, each by-product of energy metabolism has significance to the exercising athlete.
- *Capillaries* These microscopic blood vessels are not actually part of the muscle cell. Instead, capillaries physically link the muscle with the cardiovascular system. Each muscle cell may have from three to eight capillaries directly in contact with it, depending on fibre type and training. One square inch of muscle cross-section contains 125,000 to 250,000 capillaries. The volume of blood forced through the heart's aorta (about the diameter of a heavy duty garden hose) is spread so thin among the billions of capillaries that

red blood cells must squeeze through in single file. Distributing the blood flow through such an immense network of vessels is crucial, so every individual cell maintains a supply line and waste removal system.

Our bodies are obviously highly intricate and complex. Medical and sports scientists are working to understand in greater detail the body's inner workings and how it reacts to exercise.

Endurance and strength exercises increase the demand on nutrient supply and waste removal, but also stimulate the growth of more capillaries. Endurance training improves the delivery and removal function of this fantastic network of vessels. The total number of capillaries per muscle in endurance-trained athletes is about 40% higher than in untrained persons. Interestingly, this is about the same as the difference in the amount of oxygen a person can use in a minute (VO_2 max) between well-trained and untrained people. (Average VO_2 max for 20-year-olds is about 40–48 for females and 46–60 for males.) In contrast, strength training tends to decrease the capillary:muscle fibre diameter ratio. This occurs because muscle fibres grow in diameter, but the number of capillaries essentially remains unaltered.

The Motor Unit

A motor unit is the name given to a single alpha motor neuron and all the muscle fibres it activates (or innervates). With 250 million skeletal muscle fibres in the body (give or take a few million), and about 420,000 motor neurons, the average motor neuron branches out to stimulate about 600 muscle fibres.

Interestingly, large muscles may have as many as 2,000 fibres per motor unit, while the tiny eye muscles may have only ten or so fibres per motor unit. The size of a motor unit varies considerably according to the muscle's function. Muscles with high force demands but low fine control demands (like a quadriceps muscle) are organized into larger motor units. Muscles controlling high precision movements, like those required in the fingers or the eyes, are organized into smaller motor units. The motor neuron branches into many terminals, and each terminal innervates a specific muscle fibre. The motor unit is the brain's smallest functional unit of force development control; if a motor unit comprising 600 muscle fibres in the left biceps is stimulated, all 600 of those fibres will contract simultaneously and contribute to the total force produced by the biceps. The brain cannot stimulate individual fibres one at a time. Even for our sophisticated nervous system, that would require far too many connections.

Regulation of Muscular Force

The brain combines two control mechanisms to regulate the force a single muscle produces. The first is recruitment. The motor units that make up a muscle are not recruited in a random fashion. Motor units are recruited according to the size principle. Smaller motor units (with fewer muscle fibres) have a small motor neuron and a low threshold for activation. These units are recruited first. As more force is demanded by an activity, progressively larger motor units are recruited. This has great functional significance. When requirements for force are low, but control demands are high (writing, playing the piano) the ability to recruit only a few muscle fibres gives the possibility of fine control. As more force is needed, the impact of each new motor unit on total force production becomes greater. It is also important to know that the smaller motor units are generally slow units, while the larger motor units are composed of fast twitch fibres.

The second method of force regulation is called rate coding. Within a given motor unit there is a range of firing frequencies. Slow units operate at a lower frequency range than faster units. Within that range, the force generated by a motor unit increases with increasing firing frequency. If an action potential reaches a muscle fibre before it has completely relaxed from a previous impulse, then force summation will occur. By this method, firing frequency affects muscular force generated by each motor unit.

Firing Pattern

If we try and relate firing patterns to exercise intensity, we see another pattern. At low exercise intensities, like walking or slow running, slow twitch fibres are selectively utilized because they have the lowest threshold for recruitment. If we suddenly increase the pace to a sprint, the larger fast units will be recruited. In general, as the intensity of exercise increases in any muscle, the contribution of the fast fibres will increase.

For the muscle, intensity translates to force per contraction and contraction frequency per minute. Motor unit recruitment is regulated by required force. In the unfatigued muscle, a sufficient number of motor units will be recruited to supply the desired force. Initially desired force may be accomplished with

little or no involvement of fast motor units. However, as slow units become fatigued and fail to produce force, fast units will be recruited as the brain attempts to maintain desired force production by recruiting more motor units. Consequently, the same force production in fatigued muscle will require a greater number of motor units. This additional recruitment brings in fast, fatiguable motor units. Consequently, fatigue will be accelerated toward the end of long or severe bouts due to the increased lactate produced by the late recruitment of fast units.

Specific athletic groups may differ in the control of the motor units. Top athletes in the explosive sports like Olympic weightlifting or the high jump appear to have the ability to recruit nearly all of their motor units in a simultaneous or synchronous fashion. In contrast, the firing pattern of endurance athletes becomes more asynchronous. During continuous contractions, some units are firing while others recover.

JOINTS

We now understand how the muscles effect movement. As mentioned above, the muscles themselves are attached to bones. The bones form joints with each other. Joints have an architecture that depends on their function. For instance, compare the joints at the proximal (nearest to the centre of the body) end of the arm and the leg. The hip joint is very stable for obvious reasons; it has to support the upright human body. It does not, however, have the range of motion that the shoulder has. The shoulder has to have a large range of motion because, from an evolutionary point of view, we have had to reach high and low for food, and also protect ourselves. Joints, therefore, have different actions and ranges commensurate with function, largely driven by evolutionary requirements. The price that the shoulder has to pay for the greater range of motion, however, is less stability. In sport, dislocation, where the two bones in a joint shift out of place in relation to each other, is much more common in the shoulder with its greater mobility than in the more stable hip with its restricted range of motion.

Joints are enclosed by a connective tissue 'bag', called the joint capsule, and this capsule is lined by a sheet of a substance called synovium. The latter produces the nutrient fluid for the joint, and when inflamed, as in some types of arthritis, or after trauma, produces large amounts of fluid which manifests itself as joint swelling. Where the bones meet, the ends of the bones are covered by a smooth membrane, called the hyaline cartilage. This protects the bone from the weight-bearing stresses that the joint must undergo during life, and spreads the load. Loss of the hyaline cartilage leads to degenerative changes within the joint, as there is contact between the bones in the joint, with nothing to redistribute the forces. Some joints have other structures

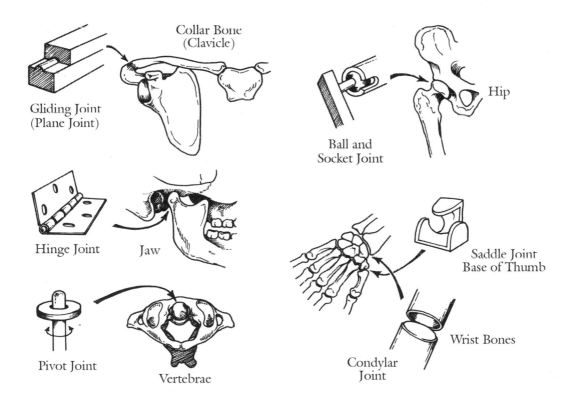

Types of joint.

35

within them which aid stability or act as extra cushioning, for instance the meniscus in the knee (which gives extra cushioning), or the rim of a similar type of material in the shoulder (which aids stability).

THE NORMAL BODY

We now have an understanding of the way the construction of the body allows movement, and how human evolution has affected development. Sport is a relatively new activity, and the most accomplished exponents are those who have inherited positive tendencies, and been able to nurture and polish these to the highest degree. That is to say that someone who would like to be a top class sportsperson would benefit from having parents with physical aptitude, and being able to train and practise would help them get the best from their physical inheritance.

There is a debate over how much exercise is healthy, and how much is too much. It is unlikely that the human body has the inherent capability to participate in the amount of sporting activity, sometimes with heavy contact, that the average professional soccer player is required to do. The strain on the body that we see today in sport has probably never before been experienced on such a wide scale – not even in the hand-to-hand combat of earlier warfare.

However, it is now evident, certainly in the Western world, that exercise is a requirement for better health. It would seem, therefore, that the medical and allied professions are obliged to help people exercise and keep healthy. By advising the exercising public, whatever their sport, on the best way to manage injuries in the early phase, and how to seek help, the

health and hence financial ramifications are inestimable.

Exercise benefits every part of the body: the heart, lungs, digestive system and even the skeleton.

THE INJURED BODY

Injuries can be divided into acute, a sudden injury such as a kick, and chronic (from the Greek *khronos* meaning 'time', but here meaning 'over a significant period of time'). Chronic injuries can further be divided into overuse injuries, where the pain is due to some repetitive strain on a part of the body, and degenerative, where injury has led to damage to an area, which may be irreversible.

Acute Injuries

Acute injuries in soccer can be caused by contact or non-contact. For example, the 'crazy horse' or dead leg is caused by local trauma to the thigh. Anterior cruciate ligament ruptures in the knee are often non-contact injuries. This type of injury is most common in senior, skeletally mature, players. However, many soccer players 'carry' ongoing injuries during play and training, which are managed day to day by medical support, and some of these injuries are chronic.

Chronic Injuries

The distinction between acute and chronic injuries may not always be cut and dried. A good way of thinking about chronic injuries are as those which 'hang around', and will not

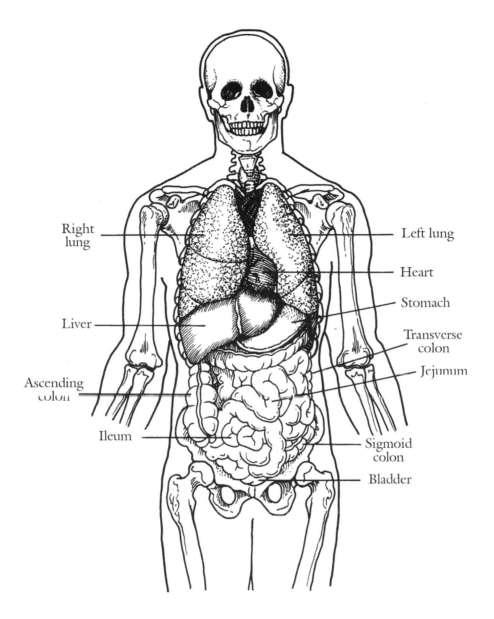

Right lung

Left lung

Heart

Stomach

Liver

Transverse colon

Jejunum

Ascending colon

Ileum

Sigmoid colon

Bladder

The internal organs.

easily settle with normal treatment. Broadly speaking, chronic injuries can be split into two groups.

Acute injuries slower to heal than normal

These are the injuries where the normal recovery period, despite treatment, is not sufficient for the injury to heal. The injury, for various reasons, refuses to settle, often prompting a review of diagnosis and patient-related factors that may affect healing.

Overuse injuries that come on slowly

These are characterized by pain associated with exercise, which comes on insidiously, and can, on occasion, prevent the player from training or playing. Often the amount or type of training can be modified to allow the player to carry on. An example of this is patellar tendonitis, an inflammation at the bottom of the patella (knee-cap), where the tendon inserts into the bone. This particular injury is often related to the player's biomechanics, and can persist even after these issues are addressed. Elite players will continue playing with this type of injury. However, if the injury is continuously irritated, there usually comes a point where training is interrupted. When this happens, the player's fitness is liable to deteriorate, and even if they play without training, performance inevitably suffers.

Deciding if, and when, the player should cease competing and enter a phase of treatment and rehabilitation can depend on the match schedule, the value of the player, and what the player wants to do. The medical team has to be sensitive to all of these factors when faced with this type of injury.

Types of Injury

Strains and sprains

Both these terms are applied to injuries of soft tissue. Strain is a more generic term and is generally applied to muscle and tendon injuries. Sprains are injuries to the ligaments. Sprains and strains are graded, denoting severity of an injury according to the percentage of muscle fibres injured. Grading gives a guide to outcome, that is, healing time, and enables a prognosis to be offered. There are three grades:

- Grade I – less than 5% of fibres
- Grade II – between 5 and 95% of fibres
- Grade III – 95% or more of fibres, which amounts, in practical terms, to a rupture.

This grading can be applied to a tendon, ligament, or muscle. The downside to this classification is its wide range: the commonest grade of tear is Grade II, which means that a player might have a 20% tear or an 80% tear, and still be diagnosed as Grade II. As stated above, grading offers a workable prognosis, but there are occasions when healing time is difficult to predict because of the lack of specificity of this grading system. The system is, at present, hard to improve upon, as the imaging techniques used in sport are not yet sophisticated enough to assess accurately the amount of damage sustained. This will change. The speed of improvement in diagnostic machines is fast, and when a more accurate grading system is employed, there will be commensurate accuracy in prognoses.

Contusions or bruises

When direct trauma is applied to any area of the body, as with a kick, tissues bleed. This is a contusion. The blood leaks from fractured small blood vessels into the surrounding structures. If viewed, there would be a pink-red hue caused by the presence of the blood. This is a bruise. Blood usually finds its way to the skin, and stains or discolours it, causing a bruise on the skin. As the blood products break down, the colour of the bruise changes as the oxygen is used; the area colour changes from a red or pink hue to a more bluish colour, before finally disappearing. A 'black eye' is an example.

CHAPTER 4

Off the Field Prevention of Injury

INTRODUCTION

Over 40 million amateurs around the world play team soccer. With 647,368 reported injuries occurring between 1989 and 1992, the risk of injury during the playing of soccer is evident. Lower extremity injuries have been found to comprise over 50% of the total injuries in soccer. Soccer injuries may be acute (e.g. sprained ankle, pulled hamstring or concussion) or chronic (e.g. overused knee, lower leg and foot problems or slow developing brain injuries). Injuries of both types can often be prevented or their incidence reduced. This may require:

- the development of more strength, flexibility and conditioning
- the use of bracing, taping or protective orthotic devices or
- changes in the rules of soccer.

Early specialization in sports can lead to overuse injuries peculiar to that one sport. Heading and knee problems in soccer, shoulder injuries in baseball, knee and ankle problems in basketball, and shoulder problems in swimming are such examples. Parents should be aware that pain in their children should be treated and that periodic absence from sport is often advisable.

A number of factors can contribute to being susceptible to injury. Older players are at greatest risk for injury, with the risk increasing about 10% per year for each year played. In the case of hamstring injuries the odds of being injured increase about 40%. Players with a previous hamstring injury have eleven times more chance of again suffering one, and for previous groin pulls there is seven times more chance of experiencing another. Players with a previous knee injury are 4.5 times more likely to experience another one and with sprained ankles the chances rise to five times (Arnason *et al.*, 2004).

It can be estimated that, on average, every élite male soccer player incurs approximately one performance-limiting injury each year. Several prevention hypotheses have been suggested, such as balance and strength programmes and ankle bracing. These seem to be particularly important in preventing the recurrence of an injury, but they may also prevent a first time injury (Junge and Dvorak, 2004).

Soccer injuries, the common cold, road traffic accidents: why is it that the universal misconception that 'it will never happen to me' rules over 'better safe than sorry'? People do get killed in traffic accidents; most people catch colds. And some players do sprain an ankle and cost their team a championship because they cannot play. Some years ago an American professional football player refused to wear hip pads: they were not required equipment back then. He was fast and shifty. He was an all-star. Then one day he was tackled with a hard contact to his hip which broke it. It ended his career and gave him a permanent disability.

Many injuries can be prevented or their severity lessened, but it may require a change in our traditional thinking. The next section looks at what might be done to prevent or reduce the more common injuries in soccer.

INJURY PREVENTION

In general the approach to safety in sport has been for the short term rather than the long term. In the past, the attitude has often been that a player who is able to play, should play, regardless of whether making an injury worse may have a negative effect on health later on in life.

In the UK, as in other countries, there have been reports on the 'occupational health' of current and retired soccer players. The surveys in the UK found that a large number of ex-professional players suffer from various ailments such as arthritis. Some cases of mental impairment in later life have been put down to excessive heading of a ball, especially when the old-fashioned leather ball was wet and therefore much heavier. So it is primarily up to the administrators of the game to afford protection by looking at the way the game is played, changing rules when necessary.

Prevention Awareness Programmes

Would it help prevent injury to explain to players how they occur? This was the subject of an Icelandic study in 2000, where players from top teams were divided, and one half saw a video programme based on injuries selected from the previous soccer season. The results showed that there was absolutely no difference between the teams that had the educational programme and those that did not (Arnason *et al.*, 2005).

A wider prevention programme has better results. Researchers from FIFA studied 194 players in seven teams that took part in a prevention programme and seven that did not. The incidence of injuries in the groups that worked specifically to prevent injuries was 21% lower. The greatest reduction of injuries was in overuse injuries and injuries occurring during practice.

Youth players also benefit from awareness training. In one study of youth players who had an awareness training course, the intervention group had 20% fewer total injuries and 30% fewer overuse injuries. It was also found that there were more injuries early in the year and that the lower-skilled players suffered more injuries – especially overuse injuries, mild injuries and injuries suffered early in the training programme. In the lower-skilled group that had the injury prevention training there were 54% fewer mild injuries but there was no reduction in the severe injuries. Match injuries were more difficult to prevent.

Recommendation

It seems that some awareness of the possible injuries should be recommended. The importance of preventative measures (which will be suggested in the chapters which follow) and other precautions should be enumerated to players, and if they are young, to their parents also. Coaches should be particularly aware of the ways that injuries can be prevented or minimized.

Intervention strategies to prevent soccer injuries can include some basic physiology related to why the players need to be strong and flexible (including a programme for accomplishing this – *see* Chapter 12) and why they need to warm-up correctly. It also helps to make players aware of the types of overuse injuries they can develop, such as Osgood–Schlatter disease for youth and turf toe and shin splints for older players. We should also make them aware of the importance of ankle injury prevention through proper bracing. The development of strong musculature in the neck and hamstrings can also be stressed. Additionally, since foul play is a major cause of injuries, an understanding of the rules and the principles of fair play should be stressed.

MEDICAL SCREENING OR PROFILING

Screening has an important role in preventive treatment of disease by targeting high risk populations for early signs of, for instance, breast cancer. The expense of screening is outweighed by the benefits of early treatment. Similarly, some soccer injuries can be prevented or reduced by soccer-specific screening. Screening soccer players' musculo-skeletal systems as a means of injury prevention requires that:

- the condition has a recognizable early phase and early treatment can be shown to improve prognosis
- effective treatment is possible and available
- the test for the condition should be rela-

tively simple, not harmful and acceptable to the patient
- the test should achieve a balance between false positives and false negatives, which is related to the severity of consequences of wrong diagnosis both for the health care system and the patient
- screening must be sustainable once introduced and not just part of a limited specific initiative.

Any debate about screening should be based around these rules of screening. As things stand, we do not know of any one musculo-skeletal factor that will prevent injury if 'treated' before the onset of symptoms. When seeing and treating injured soccer players, it is often evident that there are various factors in their physical make-up that may have predisposed them to their injury. However, it is also evident that the musculo-skeletal system acts in a concerted way, making it difficult to work out exactly how a supposed cause is actually responsible for the injury. In the absence, therefore, of a 'recognizable early phase and early treatment (that) can be shown to improve prognosis' we may have to establish a benchmark for each player, a profile of the physical and musculo-skeletal system before any injury occurs. This will be the *profile* to re-establish after the player has sustained an injury and rehabilitated from it.

The benchmark profile might be made at pre-season camp, and made annually. The rehabilitation therapist and player could thereby aim for a realistic end point that would coincide with a return to fitness. For instance, if a player sustains an uncomplicated ankle sprain, the rehabilitation should be straightforward, and the flexibility in and around the joint should be similar to that of the un-injured side (if it has not been previously injured). However, it may be that the ankle was always short on stretch, and the athlete performed perfectly well with it as it was. If the player and rehabilitation therapist are not aware of this, their rehabilitation goals may be unrealistic, and the return to play delayed. So, as things stand, screening may be unrealistic and inaccurate. However, profiling seems to be easy, practical and accurate if a strict protocol is followed, with a single person doing the measurements to avoid errors.

It is easier to apply the rules of screening in the case of disease. Intervention in the natural history of conditions with known outcomes is the aim of the medical establishment. This is generally called treatment. In soccer, medical screening is much more straightforward. A general medical examination, with blood tests and cardiac screening, should ideally be undertaken. In the UK, all young people entering the professional ranks undergo cardiac screening. The aim is to prevent sudden death on the field of play. An ECG/EKG tracing and an echocardiogram is done. The downside of this process is that not all problems are detectable by this screening. Some heart problems are extremely difficult or even impossible to detect on any screening. Those few which cannot be detected may well result in the tragic death of the young or middle-aged athlete. Pete Maravich, a top basketball player in the USA, played for many years without knowing he had only one coronary artery instead of the normal three. Years after his playing career was over he died while playing basketball with his friends at the park.

Head injuries used to be a bane of soccer. These days, there are psychometric tests that profile players. If a head injury is sustained, the physician can re-test the player and compare the profile score with the post-injury scores. Serial measurements can then be made, and a careful return to play can be managed.

Players, particularly females, should probably be measured for quadriceps:hamstring strength and the ratios of their comparison and also for a hyperextension of their knees (*genu recurvatum*). The typical quadriceps:hamstring ratio that is accepted is that the hamstrings be 60% (0.6) as strong as the quadriceps. The National Football League in the USA has adopted a ratio where the hamstrings are 75% (0.75) as strong as the quadriceps. However the ratio varies with the angle of the knee from 0.3 to 1.0 for different athletes.[1]

Recommendations

A medical case history should be completed, noting particularly a history of concussions, of muscle problems and ligament sprains, and any inherited potentials for heart problems. Minimally a doctor should listen to the heart, checking for heart murmur and any irregular heart beat. For older boys there should be a check for inguinal hernia. A secondary level of screening might be to check the relative strengths of the hamstrings to the quadriceps – aiming for at least a 7:10 ratio.

1 Conventional standards are that the hamstrings should be 0.5 to 0.6 as strong as the quadriceps at 50 degrees, from 0.4 to 1.1 for various athletes at 40 degrees (conventional standards are 0.6 to 0.7) and 0.4 to 1.4 for various athletes at a 30 degree angle (conventional standards are 0.6 to 0.8) (Aagaard *et al.*, 1998). So the optimal dynamic strength for the hamstrings should probably be generally higher than the traditional 0.6 ratio if we are to reduce the number and severity of hamstring strains.

PITCH OR FIELD

Most fatal injuries in soccer seem to occur because of a collision with the goalposts. Appropriate padding of the posts should reduce these fatalities and other injuries caused by such contact. Dr Janda and his associates at the Institute for Preventative Sports Medicine at the University of Michigan studied special padding for the goalposts and found a reduction of impact force of 31 to 63%. They then studied over 400 games where the padding was used and found no injuries when the players hit the padded posts (Janda *et al.*, 1995).

Recommendation

Pad the posts with a highly absorbent sponge type of material.

KIT OR UNIFORM

Sport is, in part, a fashion business and one in which the design of kit or uniform changes continually. In soccer, boots or shoes have become as lightweight as sprinter's spikes, with new materials taking the place of the traditional leather, which when wet became sodden and heavy. Some of the newer materials, whilst having obvious advantages, may not afford as much protection as leather.

Recommendations

To date there have been no studies on whether certain shoes will reduce ankle or knee injuries or whether the holding that is so commonly done in élite-level soccer contributes to injuries. If holding is a negative factor, very tight shirts could be worn.

COACHING AND TRAINING

Coaches and trainers have a large part to play in injury prevention. These people have a responsibility to deliver players to the start of a match in peak condition, both mentally and physically, in order to get the best result. A lot of the preparation is done on the training field, and each coaching organization will have its own approach as to what is the best way to achieve the most desirable outcome. From a physical point of view, if players are tired from doing too much training, and too near a game, this will leave them open to injury, especially late on in the game when fatigue sets in. Equally so is the situation where the player is not fit enough to match the pace of the game because of a lack of training, or the aerobic and anaerobic capacities are insufficient for the level of competition in a particular match.

Mentally, if players are 'over psyched' before a game, they may cause injury by tackling in an over-zealous way, causing injury to themselves or to opposing players. If there is suboptimal mental stimulation before a game, players can be more prone to getting injured. Getting the physico-mental preparation right is as much about experience as training, and this experience in itself is not just time spent as a coach, but knowing the players. In élite soccer, the work happens daily, and familiarity comes easily. With recreational soccer familiarity takes longer, when there may only be one training session per week, and one game.

Recommendations

Muscle strain injuries could be reduced by increased effectiveness in training methods, such as strength, power, balance and speed training, particularly in the pre-season, but continuing through the playing season. Coaches and trainers should have a knowledge of sport psychology to help them become more aware of proper levels of arousal and how to present their programmes in a manner that is more easily learned and less harassing to the players. Education updates could be forwarded through e-mail or post to keep the trainers current on scientific studies that might positively influence the safety of the game through better techniques.

LACK OF FITNESS

Coaches and medical support teams should pay more attention to jump and power training, as well as preventive measures and adequate rehabilitation of previous injuries to increase team success. This was the conclusion of the study of the top teams in Iceland (Arnason *et al.*, 2005). A significant relationship was found between team average jump height (counter-movement jump and standing jump) and team success. The same trend was also found for leg extension power, and body composition (percentage of body fat). The figures were constant for field players but goalkeepers were somewhat different, being more flexible in the knees and hips, with greater leg extension power but lower levels of conditioning, as shown by their oxygen uptake.

Strength and power activities were included in the warm-up programme by 120 teenage handball teams, both male and female, in a Norwegian study. It looked at the effects of using a warm-up programme that included a cardiovascular warm-up with strength and power activities, combined with balance and technique skills (Olsen *et al.*, 2005). Ankle and knee injuries were reduced by 50%.

Extra hamstring strength and power exercises were used in a Swedish study of thirty élite players in which half received extra hamstring strength and power exercises, largely eccentric, and the other half did not. This resulted in three injuries to the training group but ten injuries to the control group (Askling *et al.*, 2003). The training took place one to two times a week for ten weeks in addition to their normal practice time. There was also a significant increase in strength and speed to the group that received the extra training.

There is also evidence from a US study of 300 teenage female soccer players (Heidt *et al.*, 2000). Forty-two of these players participated in a seven-week training programme before the start of the season. In all injuries to the lower extremity the trained group had a significantly lower level of injuries than did the untrained group, especially ACL injuries.

Recommendations

A four-week pre-season conditioning programme might be required in which strength, flexibility and endurance could be improved – without the use of a ball.

FOUL PLAY AND RULES VIOLATIONS

Foul play is an important cause of injury in football. Reduction of foul play and adherence to the laws of the game are interventions

45

that might reduce the rate of injuries. Using videotapes of 174 professional soccer matches in which injuries occurred as a result of foul play, a panel of three FIFA referees reviewed the on-field decisions of the match referee. The panel agreed 85% with the on-field referees (Andersen *et al.*, 2004b). Another study aimed to assess:

- whether match injuries to footballers occurred as a result of players' noncompliance with the rules of the game
- whether match referees could reliably identify the legality of incidents leading to injury, and
- whether the rules of football were adequate to protect players from injury.

Using videotapes of twelve FIFA tournaments, two panels of referees judged the legality of the incidents that resulted in injury. There were 148 general injuries and 84 head or neck injuries. The match referees identified 47% of the general injuries as fouls and the expert panels identified 69% as fouls. The decisions made on the legality of tackles leading to injury indicated that the current rules of football were adequate for the majority of tackle situations, although the reliability with which referees could identify fouls during some match conditions was low. For incidents leading to head and/or neck injuries, the match referees and the referees' panel both identified a smaller proportion of injury situations as fouls (Fuller *et al.*, 2004a).

In the World Cup of 2002 a large proportion of the injuries were caused by foul play. FIFA therefore concluded that 'increased awareness of the importance of fair play may assist in the prevention of injury' (Junge *et al.*, 2004b).

Player error in tackling, often resulting in a foul, is a major cause of injuries (*see* the section 'Tackling' in Chapter 2).

Recommendations

The evidence suggests there is some reason to look at the laws of the game regarding tackling. Perhaps additional referees should be employed to be able to see more of the playing field effectively. In professional basketball (NBA) the number of officials was increased from one to two, and then to three – to watch only ten players. In American football the number of officials at the professional level has increased from four to seven, with the possibility of video viewing on the field of certain referee's decisions. Perhaps FIFA should look at the angle or mode of tackling, and if it finds the need, increase the penalties

Medical equipment for matches

First aid equipment

A professional first aid case should be available at all training sessions and matches

For treating wounds: 1½ inch training tape; 1, 2 and 4 inch roller bandages; wound cleansing wipes; vinyl gloves; antiseptic spray; assorted sticking plasters; sterile swabs; sterile dressings; double-sided non-adhesive dressings

For slowing swelling: instant ice packs; ice; freeze spray; 2, 4 and 6 inch elastic wraps; 2 and 4 inch elastic tape

For immobilizing a joint: triangular bandage, splints (inflatable, bendable aluminum, wood, etc.)

For breathing: airways, Ambu bag

for tackles that have a higher propensity for causing injury.

Dr Thor Andersen of the Oslo Sports Trauma Research Center concludes that 'the most promising strategy to reduce the risk of football injuries would be more specific wording of The Laws of the Game'. He recommends stricter penalties, and a ten-minute expulsion from the game for tactics that have a high propensity for causing injuries, such as elbowing and dangerous tackling. This expulsion might be in addition to a yellow card.

CHAPTER 5
Preventing and Reducing Head Injuries

Head injuries in soccer can occur from heading the ball, from players' heads colliding, from heads coming in contact with objects like goalposts and from blows to the head from arms or lower extremities. It is the heading that concerns most medical authorities. While we often concern ourselves with concussions from a single hard blow to the head, it is the repetitive relatively minor head traumas that are now a concern.

Acute head injuries account for between 10% and 13% of all soccer injuries, with concussions accounting for 20% of those. It may be that repeated heading of the soccer ball is one cause of head injury. Controversy exists about the possibility of neuro-cognitive impairment being caused by soccer heading. Some studies have reported that repeated heading results in a decrease in memory, planning, and IQ test scores, whereas others have reported no decrease in neuro-cognitive test scores. Improper heading technique has been associated with headaches and in some cases amnesia in 32% to 43% of players. Researchers have attributed a significant increase in the impact force when improper technique is used, which could be how the injuries are caused. It is worse for young players: improper heading technique, inexperience and skeletal immaturity may increase head accelerations, putting children at a greater risk of sustaining head injuries in soccer.

As we saw in Chapter 2, the major concern for head injuries may not be the acute concussive blow but rather the chronic sub-concussive blows from hundreds or thousands of headings. It is the blows to the head, both concussive and non-concussive, that may be a real danger to our mental functioning. Ligament sprains, muscle strains and broken bones all heal, but head injuries may alter one's human capabilities permanently. This should be our real concern.

Studies in soccer take several forms. Some look exclusively for concussive-level blows and compare the forces absorbed by boxers' heads. Other studies look at the possible problems from repeated blows to the head, which do not appear in the injury frequency charts.

THE FORCE ABSORBED BY THE HEAD

The amount of force with which the head hits an object, or vice versa, is a major factor in determining whether the brain will suffer a concussion. A 170lb (78k) player running at full speed, then losing his balance and crashing his head into a goalpost, forces his head to absorb a large number of foot/pounds of force. On the other hand, a youth size ball kicked at 30mph (50km/h), then headed, forces the head to absorb a relatively low

48

number of foot/pounds of force. Deaths from head injuries are far more likely to occur in the first instance. In terms of death rates, soccer is very safe. There are few immediate cases of an acute trauma causing death.

There is not much at this time that can be done to reduce the random head trauma due to being kicked or having a collision of heads. However, the most common blow to the head occurs during heading. There are two issues here:

- how much force a person's head can absorb before it experiences an acute trauma and a concussion
- what number of sub-concussive blows, which may lead to neurological or mental problems, can be absorbed.

There is some evidence on both issues from players with a history of heading the ball.

Most people had assumed that a force applied to the front of the head would force the brain forward, and then it would rebound back. But injuries to the brain from a blow to the front of the head seem to be worse on the back of the brain. It now appears that when a blow is struck to the front of the head the heavier spinal fluid moves forward forcing the brain backwards first. It then rebounds forward.

SPEED AND POWER OF THE BALL

The problem with summarizing all the information on ball force is that investigators use different measurements of force: newtons, foot-pounds, G (gravity) forces, and three different force scales are common measurements. But they cannot be compared well because the weight and speed of the body or ball and the

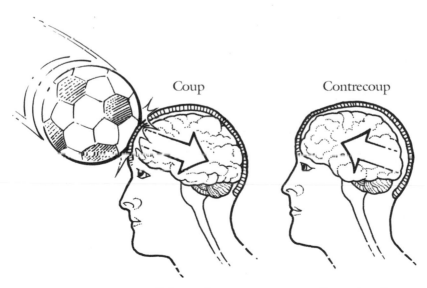

Brain movement when force is applied.

amount of movement of the head from the force of the ball all vary the measurement.[2] Consequently the relative forces found in the different studies must be compared only with similar measures.

The speed of the ball depends on the speed of the foot as it contacts the ball plus the rebound effect when the compressed ball rebounds off the foot. When skilled senior soccer players perform maximal kicks their foot velocity is on average 20.1 metres per second (m/s) but the velocity of the ball as it leaves their foot is 27.4 m/s (98.6km/h or 61mph). The fact that the ball increases in velocity after being kicked is due to the rebounding of the compressed ball off the foot. Since on a hard kick a player's foot will depress the ball considerably, the rebound from that depression at the end of the kick will increase its speed. To kick more accurately and to put spin on the ball, kickers will kick at only 80% or less than their maximum velocity (Asami *et al.*, 1976).

A soccer ball weighs 14–16oz (396–453g) and has an inflated pressure of 14.7lb/sq in (about 1kg/ sq cm, or 1 atmosphere at sea level). It can travel at speeds of 37–74mph (60–115km/h) or more. A ball kicked from 11yd (about 10m) at about three-quarter power travels at 52mph (85km/h) and strikes with an impact of 116 kilopnds (kp) or 252 foot-pounds. At full power, impact is estimated at 440 foot-pounds (200kp). Contact with the ball lasts from 1/128 to 1/63 second. Traditional leather balls can increase in weight up to 20% when wet, though this is not an issue with modern synthetic balls. A soccer ball striking the head has less impact than a typical boxing punch, producing a head acceleration of 20Gs (forces of gravity) as against 50–100Gs or more for a punch. However, a good boxer will try to slide the punch while

the soccer player may attempt to absorb the whole force in redirecting the ball. At other times the soccer player only slightly redirects the ball so does not absorb the total force of the ball. But even this type of force might send the brain crashing against the skull. More research is needed on how much of the force of the ball is absorbed by the head during different angles of redirection of the ball.

Another way to compare the force of the ball on the head is with a karate punch, which is estimated to deliver about 70–330 foot-pounds (100–450 Joules). A university group estimated the power of a punch of boxer Rocky Marciano at 1,000 foot-pounds. Others have estimated that a boxer's blow would be about 50Gs – depending, of course, on the size and speed of the boxer. A karate expert will hit and recover while maintaining balance, but a boxer will try to step into the punch with his entire weight following through. So a boxer's punch should have a greater force than a karate punch.

The mean peak forces recorded for a headed ball approach 1,000 newtons, which is less than the peak contact force produced by a professional boxer. This value is approximately half the estimated maximal peak force transmitted by a boxer's punch. This difference in impact forces may suggest that heading a soccer ball at 35mph (56km/h) does not pose the same risk as receiving a boxing punch (Broglio *et al.*, 2003).

2   Head forces are traditionally measured in 'forces of gravity' (g or G) (9.8 metres per second per second or 32 feet per second per second), SIs (severity index) or HIP (head impact power index), Joules (0.735 foot/pounds), kilopnds (kilograms of force), foot-pounds (one pound falling one foot, 1.35 Joules) and Newtons (N) (1kg per metre per second). The first two consider only the lineal speed of the implement to the head (ball or fist) while the latter also includes the rotational effect of the implement to the head. It is not possible to change all of them into one measurement.

If we look at forces of gravity (G) we find that the body can absorb possibly 300G (300 times the body's weight). Low-level brain trauma may be possible at as little as the 10–50G level of impact. Concussions have been found to occur in the 80G range but generally at 400–700G. Above 700G we expect permanent brain damage.

On a jet ski or rollercoaster ride travelling at 35mph (56km/h) on a 25-foot radius the body would be experiencing about 3G of force. With the radius shortened to 10 feet it would double the gravitational force (G). A car crash at 35mph (56km/h) would exert 35G on the body. But just plopping down in a chair might give a force of 10G.

This does not mean that accelerations over 50G always cause permanent brain damage. American football players are subjected to 30–100G, and Indy race car drivers have been subjected to 80G without permanent injury, but *they were wearing helmets*. Football players and race car drivers also protect their heads from whiplash.

Whiplash seems to be particularly damaging to the brain because the head moves a number of degrees from the vertical very quickly, bouncing the brain within the skull and causing additional damage. American football players protect against whiplash by working very hard on developing neck muscle strength and size. Many also wear a 'collar' that limits the backward movement of the head. Racing car drivers, of course, have head restraints.

Falling on the field can give a significant level of Gs. In a recent study a device was dropped from four feet above a playing field and the number of Gs absorbed was 246 for a grass field and 183–261 for various types of artificial turf (Naunheim *et al.*, 2002). Of course grass fields can vary in their absorption ability depending on the softness of the soil, the length of the grass and the moisture in the soil. So the type of field may also be a factor in the amount of force a head will absorb if a player had been airborne.

Estimates of the number of times a soccer player heads a ball vary: different sources claim an average of five per game (making 350 per year in a 70-game season); 2,000 in 300 games; and 9 times per practice and 7 times per game. European players seem to head the ball more frequently than other players.

When the kicked ball contacts the head, the impact on the head will depend on several things:

- the mass of the head (how much the head weighs)
- how stiff the neck was and how strong were the neck muscles (a stiff neck will allow the whole body to absorb the force of the ball), and
- the speed and weight of the ball.

The larger a child's head, the less movement is generated when a ball hits it. Also the larger the ball the more force to the child's head. So children should not be allowed to play with balls larger than that acceptable for their age.

Concussions

Concussions occur when a blow to the brain is sufficient to do immediate damage to brain functions, such as unconsciousness, dizziness or inability to think clearly. The amount of force necessary to cause a concussion depends on a number of factors:

- genetics
- the part of the skull that is hit
- the force of the blow
- the length of time it takes for the blow to be absorbed (a blow to a helmeted head may take milliseconds longer to affect the brain because the time that the force is being applied is lengthened as it is absorbed in the cushioning material, thereby reducing its severity)
- the amount of movement of the head due to the force (which is reduced when the neck is stiffer and the body absorbs more of the force of the blow)
- a history of previous concussions.

Elite soccer players have a 50% chance if male, and 22% if female, of sustaining a concussion while playing soccer over a ten-year period (Barnes *et al.*, 1998). A player who has had one concussion is in greater danger of repeated concussions. A player who has had three concussions is nine times more likely not only to have more, but also to suffer more negative effects from them. This gives weight to the assertion that repeated head traumas will have cumulative effects.

Studies conducted on animals have shown that concussion is induced with difficulty when the head is held in a fixed position but more easily when the head is allowed to move freely. Woodpeckers smack their heads against trees with 1200G of force without suffering brain damage, partly because they keep their heads in the plane of their body (i.e. have a stiff neck); the head does not rotate up and down or right and left during the pecking. This is the reason that strong neck muscles and a rigid body are more protective against concussions when heading.

Any player with dizziness, headache or neck pain after heading a ball should be evaluated for a mild concussion. Usually this just requires removing the player from the game, but repeated complaints need to be seriously considered for medical evaluation.

Repetitive Sub-concussive Blows

Heading is often compared with boxing or with American football in that the participants may receive a number of blows at sub-concussive level but that these blows may have cumulative effects. Well over fifty years ago the sport researcher Ernst Jokl found that the accumulation of blows to boxers' heads tended to show injuries where there was a rough area at the juncture of the various skull bones. Each blow would cause what Jokl called a 'pinpoint haemorrhage', which tended to be found in different spots in different boxers. If the rough area was in the rear of the skull, where vision is registered, there could be vision problems; if it was on the right side of the skull, the parietal area, there would likely be sensory (feeling) or motor (movement) problems on the boxer's left side. If the area affected was in the front of the brain, memory problems were likely.

There is no conclusive evidence to settle the controversy surrounding the idea that repeated trauma from heading the ball can cause a cumulative brain injury similar to that seen in boxers. A number of attempts have been made to research the question, with active and retired soccer players serving as both the focus of study and as controls. A number of methods have been used to evaluate brain damage and brain function in these studies.

Electro-encephalography

Evaluation of brain traumas using the electro-encephalograph (EEG) allows the investigator to check the electrical output of various parts of the brain. It can give a picture of where a brain is normal or abnormal. Tysvaer and Storli used a neurologic and electro-encephalographic (EEG) approach in their study of 69 active Norwegian first division soccer players (aged 15–34), ten of whom considered themselves to be typical headers, and a control group of 69 age-matched men with no history of neck or head injury and no soccer experience. The results showed that abnormal EEGs were more numerous among players than among controls. Abnormal EEGs were more common in younger players, which the authors attributed to a greater susceptibility to trauma, skeletal immaturity, or possibly less experience and skill.

Another EEG study reported neurological and neuropsychological test results in 53 former champion amateur boxers and 53 former first division soccer players. Slight symptoms were found in 45% of boxers and 70% of the soccer players, especially involving concentration or memory impairment (Thomassen et al., 1979). One study looking at brain damage in boxers used soccer players and track athletes as controls. EEG abnormalities were seen in 20% of the soccer players. This was not significantly different from boxers or track athletes. No severe EEG abnormalities were found (Haglund and Eriksson, 1993).

Computerized tomography

Computerized tomography (CT or CAT scans), which gives a three-dimensional picture of body organs was used to evaluate possible head injuries in 33 former Norwegian first division soccer players who averaged 52 years old, had played an average of 329 games and had quit playing an average of eighteen years previously. Widened brain ventricles were found in 27% of the players and 9% had questionable widening. Central and/or cortical atrophy was seen in 33%. Nine typical headers, who were significantly older, also had the highest frequency of atrophy. The authors, Sortland and Tysvaer (1989), noted that the findings on visual evaluation exceeded the frequencies observed in a study of the Danish general population.

Magnetic resonance imaging

Magnetic resonance imaging (MRI) scanning was used to look for brain injuries in a study comparing twenty members of the US national soccer team (average age 24.8 years) with twenty élite male track-and-field athletes (average age 26.4 years). The investigators, Jordan et al. (1996), also used a heading frequency index and symptom reports; they found that only prior acute head injury correlated with symptoms reported by players. No relationship was found between heading and severity of symptoms. Forty-five per cent of soccer players had abnormal MRI findings, including cortical atrophy, focal atrophy and cavum septum pellucidum (CSP), and 30% of controls had comparable findings. The incidence of CSP in the US soccer team was 15%, exceeding the 1% typically found in the general population. The researchers could not rule out the possibility that heading exacerbates previous injury or that encephalopathic changes will occur later in life.

A significant number of symptoms were reported in a survey of 128 active Norwegian soccer players by Tysvaer and Storli. The athletes, who had played an average of 100 games each, reported both 'protracted' or chronic and permanent symptoms, including headache, neck pain, and dizziness. Migraine headaches have also been associated with heading.

Neuropsychological testing

Neuropsychological testing is another way to measure brain functioning. Tests ascribe an individual's functions in the range of normal, inferior or superior. Such a neuropsychological approach was used in comparing 37 former Norwegian National Team soccer players with 20 hospitalized patients as controls (Tysvaer and Lochen, 1991). Results indicated that differences between subtest scores in verbal performance were greater in soccer players than in the control group (scores on the verbal performance subtests are expected to be about equal). Soccer players also scored less well on other tests. Of the soccer players, 81% had some degree of neuropsychological impairment, compared with 40% of the controls. Headers had a slightly higher frequency of 'severe' or 'severe to gross' neuropsychological impairment than non-headers.

Animal research has shown that moderate repetitive blows to the skull with short time intervals cause more severe brain damage than intense blows at intervals of days or weeks (Sortland and Tysvaer, 1989). Repeated headings may not only negatively affect brain function, but may eventually be fatal. Former England World Cup striker Jeff Astle was renowned as a great header of a soccer ball. He never knew it would kill him. In what could be a groundbreaking decision, a coroner ruled that Astle died at 59 from a degenerative brain disease caused by the constant heading of a heavy and often wet soccer ball.

Despite the protection offered by correct technique and adequate conditioning, a study of four élite players (Barnes *et al.*, 1998) resulted in the reporting of headaches by all four after ten minutes of heading. In addition, it has been reported that half of the Olympic soccer players studied had at least one headache after heading; they also reported the worsening of headaches with exertion, throbbing headaches, and bilateral symptoms. The players typically ascribed symptoms to poor heading technique.

Helmet Evaluation

Should helmets be used in soccer? It has been suggested, but is unlikely to be adopted, both because of tradition and the feeling that heading directly on the skin gives better control. In addition, helmet use may not effectively diminish acceleration-type injuries: helmets do not eliminate total impact but rather spread the absorption of that impact over more milliseconds as the foam absorbs the force.

Conclusions

While the research is not conclusive, most of the evidence suggests that playing soccer, probably with heading as a major factor, may increase the chances of decreased mental performance and brain-related ailments. However, research needs to be better controlled in terms of the variables considered and the possible causes of brain damage or neurological complications (e.g. memory problems, headaches). Other variables to consider that might have caused brain problems are excess alcohol intake, auto accidents with accompanying whiplash, fighting, or playing other sports that might have caused minor brain injury.

Recommendations

What can be done now to reduce the severity of blows to the head by the ball is to strengthen the muscles of players in the front and sides of the neck. In this way, the force of the ball is not entirely absorbed by the rocking of the head back with the ensuing bouncing of the brain inside the skull. With the muscles strongly contracting as the ball meets the head, some of the force of the blow will be absorbed by the whole body. Neck strengthening exercises are explained in Chapter 12.

Heading technique can also be improved to reduce the movement of the head as it contacts the ball. The body's movement should be slowed if possible, the ball should be hit with the front part of the head rather than the side of the head, which results in fewer injuries, and the neck must be stiff.

Another factor that can reduce head injuries is to eliminate the use of the arms and hands above the shoulders. With effective rules, and their enforcement, injuries to the head by an opponent's arms or hands can be minimized.

Younger children should play without heading the ball. If heading continues to be allowed this skill should be reserved for older, stronger players.

While designing an acceptable helmet would make sense, players and administrators are not yet ready for such a radical departure from tradition. If a reduction of bruises and some skull fractures is the goal then a sponge type of helmet such as worn by some rugby players may suffice. But if nearly complete protection against skull fractures and a huge reduction of recurrent trauma is the goal then an American football helmet is necessary. These have a hard shell with air and foam padding and special suspensions that will soften and redistribute the blows. Present soccer headgear does not reduce the total impact on the head, it just spreads it out over more milliseconds. However, this may be all that is needed to somewhat reduce the whiplash effect that is a major cause of brain injury.

The clinical effectiveness of soccer headbands remains to be seen. With peak forces of 1,000 newtons or less but for hundreds of headings per season, perhaps effective headgear has the potential to minimize brain damage. Headbands decrease the effect of the impact because of their cushioning effect. The thicker or more absorbent the cushioning material, the longer it takes from initial contact with the material to the absorption of the blow by the skull. The power of a boxer's punch takes longer to register on the head than does a soccer ball because of the thickness of the glove on the hand. However, because headbands have a lower peak impact force than none at all, they decrease the total effect of impact over the same time when compared with using none. The thicker the absorbing material the less impacting force on the head.

EYE INJURIES

There has been some research in this area. Soccer balls projected at 18mps were found to penetrate about ¼in (8mm) into the eye socket. The ball remains on the eye socket for a hundredth of a second and seems to have a suctioning effect as it leaves. This could pull the eye forward past its normal resting place after it had been compressed, possibly causing damage. Those who studied this (Vinger and Capao, 2004) recommended the use of protective eyewear.

Recommendations

Without protective goggles it is not easy to prevent eye injuries. Players who have better peripheral awareness may be able to avoid them. The relatively new field of sports vision can train peripheral vision, and this may, in the future, be part of player conditioning. Otherwise, there are those who have worn hardened plastic facial protection, especially in the post-rehabilitation phase after return to play. These are not generally worn as primary prevention, however. Perhaps it should be considered.

MOUTH AND TEETH INJURIES

Mouth and teeth injuries are always a possibility in any contact sport, but soccer has nowhere near the risk that boxing or American football used to have. Boxing has, of course, required mouthguards for many years. American football players, especially the linemen, rarely had a full set of teeth before mouthguards were required. Now a dental injury is unheard of. Parents in the USA, when asked, thought that mouthguards should be used in football, especially by boys (Diab and Mourino, 1997). A study in Australia found that without a mouthguard, the likelihood of a broken or lost tooth was at least double. Some injuries occurred despite the wearing of mouthguards. During the two years of the study (Jolly *et al.*, 1996) over two seasons, mouthguard ownership and consistent wear increased and dental injuries decreased.

Recommendations

Mouthguards should be required for practice and games to reduce the chance of dental or mouth injuries. The padding between the teeth also seems to reduce the shock of a blow to the jaw that might cause a concussion or a sub-concussive brain injury.

CHAPTER 6

Preventing and Reducing Ankle and Foot Injuries

THE ANKLE

Ankle injuries are very common in sports that involve running, jumping or collisions. Soccer involves all three. Various studies have shown that the rate of ankle injuries is between 11 and 25% of all acute injuries.

The most common injuries are ankle sprains to the lateral ligaments. Some people are born with tough tight ligaments and will seldom sprain an ankle. Others are born with smaller and looser ligaments and are particularly susceptible to ankle sprains. Based on a number of studies we can expect one sprained ankle every 10–20 matches. While ankle sprains account for about 20% of all injuries, they are the most preventable: few ankle sprains need ever occur.

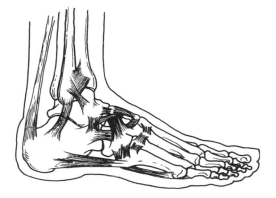

Ankle ligaments.

Injuries to the ankle are not so much the fault of the sport, but rather are due to the structural properties of the ankle joint with its multiple bones and the multiplicity of ligaments connecting them. This structure, along with the fact that it is the base of the leg that is running or jumping, makes it more susceptible to injury.

Two mechanisms, thought to be specific to football, have been identified on videotape of matches:

- player-to-player contact with impact by an opponent on the inside of the leg just before or at foot strike, resulting in an outward-directed force causing the player to land with the ankle in a vulnerable, inverted position
- forced plantar flexion (bending the ankle towards the sole) where the injured player hit the opponent's foot when attempting to shoot or clear the ball.

Prevention of Ankle Injury

The methods used to prevent ankle sprains include:

- balance training
- strengthening the ankle muscles
- wearing high top shoes

57

- taping the ankles
- using stiff cloth lace-up supports or using semi-rigid stirrup-type ankle braces.

Balance board training

Balance board training does two things. It can develop better proprioception (the sense of knowing where a part of the body is in space) and it helps slightly to strengthen the muscles in the lower leg.

Before modern stirrup braces were perfected, a Swedish study (Tropp *et al.*, 1985) showed that soccer players with no ankle protection had 17% ankle injuries (of all injuries). If they had ankle disk balance training they reduced it to 5%. With ankle braces, but no disk training, it was reduced to 3%. The conclusion was that coordination training on a balance board ought to be included in the rehabilitation of ankle injuries to prevent functional instability. It may also be done by players with previous ankle problems to help prevent further injury and therefore break the vicious circle of recurrent sprains and the feeling of 'giving way'.

Using tape on ankles

There is a long tradition of using tape to prevent spraining the ankles. In 2005, of the Arsenal team players, 60% have ankle strapping with tape and 70% of those have not had an injury that they are protecting. None of the players uses an ankle brace. So 40% play without ankle protection.

Research findings which show that taping is less effective than earlier believed are:

- athletic tape loses 40% of its initial support after ten minutes of exercise
- the skin on which the tape is applied moves, reducing its effectiveness
- tape fails to maintain a consistent amount of support for extended periods of activity, and
- perspiration limits its effectiveness.

Different kinds of ankle taping

There are two approaches to taping the ankle. One is to use the tape as a sort of a cast, which tends to immobilize the ankle. This is the more common but less effective method. The other method is to tape actively to reinforce the lateral ligaments where most ankle sprains occur.

In making the 'cast', what is generally used is 'pre-wrap' – a flimsy foam-type wrap that keeps the tape off the skin so that it is easier and less painful to remove. The tape will generally be brought only about one-third of the way up the ankle. The foot will be taped in a neutral position. The way the tape is applied is quite similar in the two types of taping, the difference is in the amount of upward pressure on the lateral side in applying the stirrups' figure eights and heel locks. In the more active reinforcing taping the tape will be applied to the skin, to reduce the amount of slippage and better protect the ligaments, and the tape will come higher up the leg to minimize the play of the skin over the muscles and bones and so support the ligaments more effectively. The foot will be turned upward to the outside.

Whichever method is chosen, use a high-quality athletic tape of one-and-a-half inch width. The Internet is a good source of adequate taping diagrams for the 'cast' taping.

What follows is a description of the more effective lateral ligament taping.

How to Tape an Ankle

The ankle should be shaved to about 12in (30cm) above the sole of the foot. Then a sticky substance such as tincture of benzoin, or a spray such as Tuffskin should be applied. Pre-wrap should not be used because it moves under the tape. Even when taping to the skin, the skin will be able to move over the joint so the tape cannot reinforce the ligament strength completely. After the spray has dried, a tape anchor or two can be wrapped around the foot just behind the foot pad at the metatarsal arch and one or two about 10–12in (25–30cm) above the sole of the foot and around the belly of the gastrocnemius.

For maximum ligament support make certain the athlete holds the ankle up and to the outside. Put a shoestring around the small toe and have the athlete pull on it to pull the outside of the foot upward. Most of the wraps will start from the inside of the foot and put upward pressure on the outside of the ankle because the tape is there primarily to support the lateral ligaments.

Starting on the inside of the leg at the anchor, run a stirrup under the foot, behind the protuberance of the fifth metatarsal bone (see below). Taping over that spot may make the foot 'go to sleep'. Pull up hard to the outside and press the tape to the skin. Use three or four such stirrups. The tape now supports the lateral ligaments and helps to prevent the ankle from turning under. Use three or four of these stirrups overlapped about a half-inch (2cm). There have been cases where two or three of the stirrups have been ripped

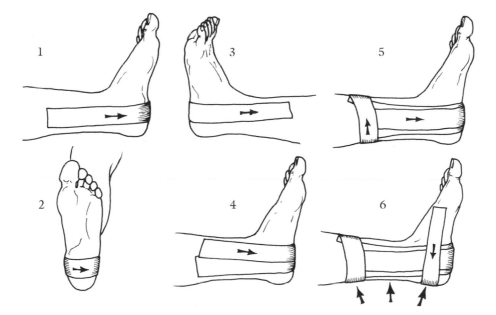

Taping an ankle: the stirrups.

crossways just over the ligament because of a strong blow that would otherwise have ripped the ligament.

Most of the rest of the tape job is to secure these stirrups and to add some additional support on both the inside and the outside of the ankle (*see* page 59).

Some tapers will use horseshoes starting from the middle of the inside of the foot around the Achilles tendon, ending on the outside of the foot next to where it started. This, while common, does not add much strength.

Next make a figure eight to hold the stirrups close to the skin. Starting just in front of the tibia at the ankle joint bring the tape under the foot on top of the stirrups, pull up to the outside, cross over the starting point and bring the tape around the back of the ankle, inside to outside, then anchor it to the starting point. Some tapers use a second figure eight starting from the outside and moving inside and around the lower leg. However, the heel lock will do the same thing so it is not really necessary.

The lateral heel lock comes next. Start with the tape in front of the lateral malleolus, go across the top of the foot, under the foot, then back around the Achilles tendon and finish about where the tape started. Next do the reverse, start in front of the medial malleolus, bring the tape to the lateral side, under the foot and angle it up and back around the Achilles tendon, then back to about where it started.

Figure eights could have been applied here or earlier. But the tape needs to be anchored with more training tape or elastic wrap. Do not leave 'bubbles' of skin that may be irritated.

Wrap several horseshoes around the upper ankle to the top of the tape job. Start in the front of the leg, wrap around one time and end at the starting place, leaving a little space between the ends so that the circulation is not cut off. The socks will help to keep the tape in place.

Ankle braces

For well over fifty years American college football players have had their ankles taped daily for practice. At secondary school level they were taped for games and usually used stiff ankle wraps for practices. Nowadays most use ankle braces daily because they are so effective.

Research has shown that braces reduce the chance of re-spraining an ankle by six times; usually a re-sprain is twice as likely as not. Ankle braces have also been shown to reduce repeated ankle injury better than taping in competitive female soccer players with a history of ankle injuries (Sharpe *et al.*, 1997).

To prevent ankle sprains the ankles should be taped or braced daily. Studies show that taping will reduce ankle sprains to some degree but that ankle braces are far more effective. Bracing can either prevent the sprain or reduce its severity. Ankle braces are absolutely recommended before a player's first sprain; they help prevent a second sprain if they were not worn soon enough. Do not buy an elastic ankle sleeve to prevent a sprain. Elastic can help to reduce the swelling after a sprain is incurred, but it does not prevent a sprain. To prevent a sprain one needs to support the ligaments in the ankle – particularly the lateral ligaments.

Braces, as far as we know, are always better than taping, with the possible exception of the first ten minutes after tape is applied. The tape

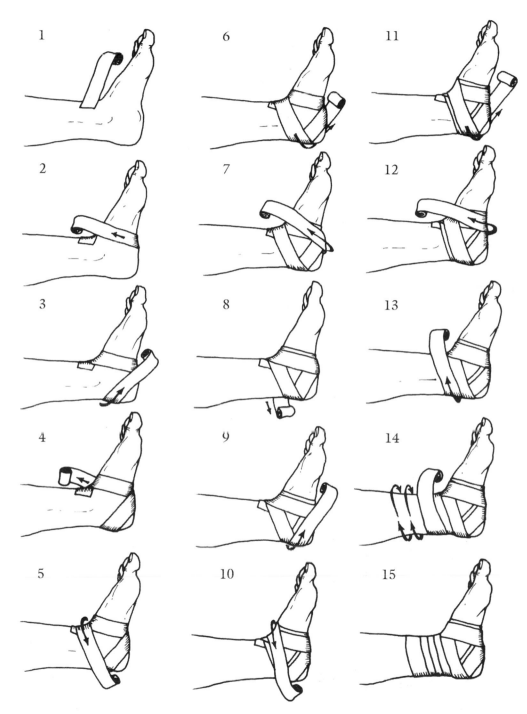

Taping an ankle: the wrap.

tends to start losing its stiff protecting qualities within 10–20 minutes after it is applied. The braces, on the other hand, maintain their protective qualities for years. They are much less expensive in the long run.

Some people think that taping or braces may offer a false sense of security and may put the athlete at greater risk for injury. No scientific evidence supports this idea.

The question that needs to be asked is which brace is better for soccer players today and whether a better brace can be developed specifically for soccer.

While some people have hypothesized that bracing would weaken the muscles around the ankle, research has not found this to be true (Cordova *et al.*, 2000). A major muscle in the area, the peroneus longus, is not negatively affected by ankle bracing. In fact bracing seems to increase the muscle's reaction time (Karlsson and Andreasson, 1992). There are other favourable findings for the muscles and the joint that indicate that bracing has only positive effects.

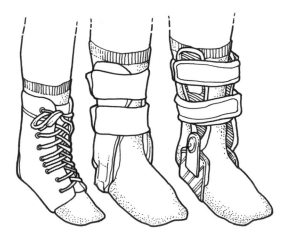

Three kinds of ankle brace: lace up, air cast and hinged.

The earliest braces were made of a thick, stiff material, sometimes reinforced on the sides for stiffness, and laced in the front. This type of brace is the least expensive, and while it does the job of reducing the possibility of an ankle sprain to some degree, it often limits the up and down motion of the foot. More recently stirrup braces have been developed which prevent the inward and outward movements (inversion and eversion) of the ankle but still allow upward and downward movement (dorsiflexion and plantar flexion). They also are generally easier to put on, and adjust, since Velcro is a common fastener. Soccer players may prefer this type of brace although it may cost 40–300% more.

Semi-rigid and laced ankle braces have significantly reduced the incidence of initial and recurrent ankle sprain injuries in both athletes and military personnel. With few exceptions, these braces do not appear to affect functional performance adversely. Additional research is needed to evaluate the many new braces that are available and in use and their influence on the incidence of ankle sprain injury and functional performance.

Braces, whether secured by laces or Velcro, may lose some of their protective advantages if they are not sufficiently secured. But braces can quickly be tightened during a practice or game if they are found to be loose.

Some players have blister problems when beginning to use the braces, which can be prevented by using moleskin or socks under the brace. When choosing a brace, remember that some are made to prevent injury while others are made to protect an already injured ankle by increasing its immobilization; avoid the latter. Use the

Internet to see what choices are available, before buying at a sporting goods store. The site epinion.com is useful in finding out about others' experience with the different braces.

Cost effectiveness of braces

Braces cost from £24 to £100 pounds each in the UK in 2005, but only $18 to $45 in the USA. As an approximate cost analysis, if both ankles were taped five days a week for four months, the cost would be about three to six times more for the tape than for a pair of braces – depending on the cost of the braces (bearing in mind what the tape cost, the cost of a trainer or therapist to apply the tape, under-wrap if used and benzoin spray.) In terms of cost effectiveness, even the older lace-up braces are only about one-sixth the cost of tape (Olmsted *et al.*, 2004).

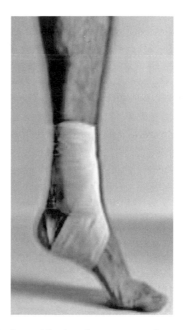

A typical tape job: the stirrups are too short.

THE FOOT

The condition called 'turf toe' is caused by the hyperextension of the big toe. It is, in effect, a sprain. It has increased over the last several years, primarily because of the increased use of artificial playing surfaces and softer, more flexible shoes (Allen *et al.*, 2004). Prevention is effected by using stiffer-soled shoes and, if possible, by not playing on artificial turf. It is possible that strengthening the muscles under the feet may help. Such exercises as curling a towel under the feet with the toes may help. A stiff insole orthotic device may also prevent this type of injury as well as reduce the chances of tendinitis in the heel and under the arches of the feet.

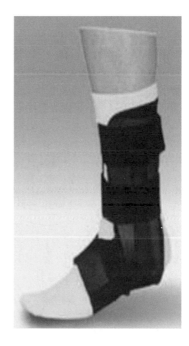

Ankle brace.

CHAPTER 7

Preventing and Reducing Other Injuries

In the previous chapters we have covered the head and the feet, which are the major areas of concern. In this chapter we will cover prevention of injuries to the rest of the body, that is, from the neck to the shin.

Each body part is susceptible to injury to some degree. The number and severity of the injuries depends on the sex and age of the player, the level of competition, and the skills that the player must execute. We will start with the feet and work upwards, pointing out the research available relative to causes and prevention of the more common injuries or problems.

ACHILLES TENDON

Achilles tendinitis, pain in the tendon above the heel, is common. Heel pain and arch pain are also common. An arch support will usually help these problems. If the Achilles tendon is sore, a quarter-inch pad can be inserted into the heel of the shoe. This will reduce the stretch on the tendon. Also, players should wear soccer boots only during games or practice.

Recommendations

If there are heel tabs (a raised tab at the back of the shoe) they can be cut off. While they were originally intended to cushion the Achilles tendon, in many people they stretch and irritate the tendon. The Achilles tendon can be stretched after practice by standing flat-footed a yard or more from a wall, then leaning forward into the wall. If a stretch is not felt above the back of the heel, move further away from the wall.

THE SHIN

One of the most serious soccer injuries is a fracture of both bones of the lower leg. The fracture is usually at a level near the top of the shin guard. It usually occurs when two players going for the ball at the same time clash. One player misses the ball and kicks the other with enough force to break both the tibia and fibula bones of the lower leg. The leg needs to be splinted and the player seen immediately by an orthopaedic surgeon. Surgery is needed for some fractures, usually those that are unstable or that break the skin.

Shin guards are used almost universally in soccer. Load forces have been shown to be reduced by 41–77% with the utilization of shin guards. This obviously reduces the number and severity of potential bruises and breaks. While they spread out the impact of a blow across the whole guard, they are not very helpful in preventing fractures. Shin guards that spread out the impact the most are the air/foam cell pads that happen to be the biggest ones on the market. Most kids want the bare minimum to pass the referee's inspection, but the reality is that the bigger the guard, the more the protection.

Shin splints are an irritation of the muscle in the front of the shin. It is an overuse injury and is most likely to occur when the athlete has been running repeatedly on a hard surface. Non-shock absorbent soles may also contribute to this condition.

Recommendations

Players should wear shin guards, which should be (and usually are) compulsory at lower levels of play. If possible play should be on grass and players should wear shoes with more absorbent cushioning in the sole, or use effective inner soles.

THE KNEE

Knee injuries are usually relatively serious. For the most part they are sprains of the knee ligaments or tears to the cartilage that protects the thighbone (femur) and lower leg bones (fibula and tibia). The risks of non-contact knee injuries include:

- laxity – loose ligaments due either to prior injury or genetics
- muscle imbalance – the quadriceps are usually significantly stronger than the hamstrings
- enervation timing – the muscles contracting at different times, a couple of milliseconds later, which stresses the tissues in the knee toward the quicker contract-

ing muscle, a more common problem in females
- general motor skills – cutting, stopping and jumping.

Any running or jumping activity, especially during body collisions, increases the chances of knee injuries. While preventative knee bracing is often used for American football linemen, they are too cumbersome and heavy to be used in soccer. The prevention of knee injuries seems to be most effectively done through appropriate strength and power training (*see* Chapter 12) and through learning appropriate cutting, landing and stopping techniques as well as balance work. This is particularly important for female soccer players (Junge and Dvorak, 2004).

Balance Training

Proprioceptive balance training has been shown to reduce the incidence of ankle sprains in different sports so it was tried as a preventative activity for knee injuries. An Italian study of 600 soccer players in forty teams (Caraffa *et al.*, 1996) looked at the possible preventive effect of a gradually increasing proprioceptive training on four different types of wobble-boards during three soccer seasons. It was found that the proprioceptively trained players had significantly fewer ACL injuries than those with none. However, a Swedish study on female players showed a contradictory outcome (Soderman *et al.*, 2000). Those receiving balance board training had four ACL injuries to one for the control group. But of those who had been injured within three months of the beginning of the study, the injury rates were lower for those who had the balance board training.

Shoe Design

Shoe design might reduce the risk of knee and lower leg injuries. Some years ago a novel idea was tried for American football shoes. The front cleat was a large circle, about two-and-a-half inches (6cm) in diameter and a half-inch (1cm) thick. The shoe unquestionably reduced knee injuries because the cleat allowed the leg to pivot when a force was applied. Perhaps such a stud might be researched for soccer.

Strength Development

According to data from the National Collegiate Athletic Association Surveillance System, knee injuries have increased among female basketball and soccer players compared with their male counterparts. A study of 53 healthy high-level collegiate athletes playing soccer, basketball or field hockey measured:

- knee hyperextension (*genu recurvatum*)
- the muscle strength ratio between the quadriceps and hamstrings (HG ratio)
- the tightness of the iliotibial band, a sheet of fibrous tissue on the outside of the thigh.

The object of the study (Devan *et al.*, 2004) was to see if any of these factors predisposed the female athletes to overuse injuries of the knee. During the playing season ten overuse injuries to the knee occurred. There were five iliotibial band friction syndrome cases,

three patellar tendonitis cases and two other complaints. It was found that those athletes with greater *genu recurvatum* and with lower hamstring strength were most likely to suffer injuries. Knee ligaments seem to tear during landing, stopping or cutting in an erect stance (straight knee and straight hip). This is especially true in females. Players, particularly girls, should play with a lower centre of gravity (the old 'athletic ready position') and absorb these shocks by flexing the hips and knees. This needs to be taught when the players are still young.

Dislocations of the knee-cap are a common soccer injury, especially in females. Braces

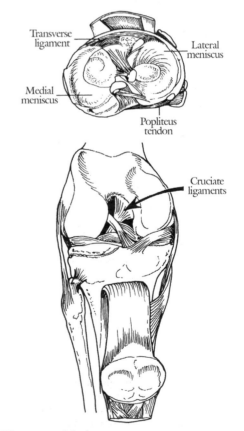

Ligaments of the knee.

or elastic sleeves with a hole for the knee-cap are sometimes used after an injury to protect the knee. Braces may also be used to prevent injury.

Anterior cruciate ligament (ACL) injuries in sport are common and most occur during non-contact cutting manoeuvres. ACL failure occurs when the ligament load exceeds its strength. In a study comparing strength training with balance training[3] it was found that the balance group performed the best in the tests of cutting, running and side-stepping. The researchers (Cochrane *et al.*, 2003) measured several factors that are believed to be preventative in reducing ACL injuries, including the inward and outward (valgus–varus) movement of the knee in cutting and stopping, and the degree that the knee was flexed when under pressure from stopping or cutting. Both of these reduce the load on the knee. While the balance group reduced the valgus–varus motion of the knee, the free weight group found an increase in this negative factor. Both the balance and the machine weight-and-balance group increased the amount of knee flexion when cutting and stopping. This should allow more of the force being absorbed to be handled by the muscles rather than being absorbed by the ACL. The free weight exercises used in the study seem to be inappropriate for knee loading movements. However it is conceivable that while the free weight work increased the knee instability in the measures used in the research, the strength gained may have

made up for this in the actuality of injury occurrence on the field. This was not measured in the study.

Recommendations

Hamstring strength needs to be increased in both males and females, but females will probably profit more from gaining such strength (*see* Chapter 12). More endurance work, both in the gym and on the field is also needed, especially for the females. It would seem advisable for both male and female athletes to strive for a hamstring strength level at least 70% of that of the quadriceps. Females also may require more fundamental skills in stopping and cutting in which they flex their knees and hips more than is commonly done. Probably effective balance training will be helpful in reducing knee injuries.

THE THIGH

For the most part thigh injuries are bruises and muscle pulls, particularly in the hamstrings. Many predisposing factors for hamstring strain have been suggested in the literature, including:

* insufficient warm-up
* poor flexibility
* muscle imbalances
* muscle weakness
* neural tension
* fatigue
* dysynergic contraction of muscle groups (not co-ordinated: different rates of contraction speed)
* previous injury.

---

3 The study used four groups: a balance training group, a free weight group, a machine weight group and a combination machine and balance group, with training sessions three times a week for thirty minutes each time and for twelve weeks.

The evidence to substantiate these speculations is minimal and conflicting. It seems also that many hamstring injuries happen during the eccentric action when the thigh is being swung forward after having completed the power phase of the running stride or in the transition from the stretching eccentric contraction to the concentric contraction as it starts its backward power movement.

A study of hamstring injuries in English professional football (Hawkins *et al.*, 2004) over two seasons involved all but one of the 92 Premier and Football League clubs. It showed that hamstring strains accounted for 12% (796 hamstring strains) of the total injuries sustained over the two seasons; 67% occurred during matches. Nearly half occurred during the last third of the first and second halves of the match. Most occurred in Premier League players (28%). Of those who experienced a hamstring strain during the year, 12% re-injured them during that year. Players were 2.5 times more likely to sustain a hamstring strain than a quadriceps strain during a game.

A similar study of 146 Belgian professional soccer players (Witvrouw *et al.*, 2003) found that the players with less flexibility in the hamstrings or quadriceps had significantly more injuries to these muscle groups. However, the same was not true for calf flexibility nor adductor flexibility for calf strains or groin pulls.

Imbalances of muscles may contribute to thigh injuries. In a study of 138 female athletes (Knapik *et al.*, 1991) it was found that there was a greater chance of a leg injury if the right hamstrings were 15% or more stronger than the left hamstrings, or if the right gluteals were 15% or more stronger than the left gluteals, or if there was a relative weakness of the hamstrings to the quadriceps of 25% or more. These data suggest that strength exercises and balancing the relative strengths of the hip and leg muscle groups is important. The earlier cited Swedish study (Askling *et al.*, 2003) strongly indicates that strength work will reduce leg injuries.

Developing Eccentric Strength

Strength in the hamstrings, particularly the eccentric strength (the strength shown while the muscle is lengthening, such as when the thigh is being brought forward during a running stride) is apparently critical to preventing hamstring pulls. This seems to be particularly true when the hamstrings are weaker than the quadriceps.

An interesting Australian study examined eccentric exercise for hamstrings to prevent muscle strains and to prevent recurrence for those who had had such injuries. It is common knowledge that hamstring strains are likely to occur during the eccentric action when the thigh is being brought forward after forcefully driving backwards in the power phase of the running stride. It was hypothesized that the normal damage done to a muscle fibre during eccentric actions might be a cause of a larger level of muscle damage when the eccentric action was particularly forceful. The researchers (Proske *et al.*, 2004) proposed that a mild regimen of eccentric exercise should be undertaken not only for those prone to re-injury but also for those who have not been injured. Such exercise has also been suggested by the Norwegian sports injury group.

Special eccentric strengthening regimes can reduce the number of hamstring pulls. A

Swedish study of two teams from their top league showed that such injuries were reduced by 66%, and that speed was increased in the trained group (Askling *et al.*, 2005). A French study compared eleven élite players who had at least one hamstring injury during the previous two years to seventeen players with none. When the eccentric (lengthening strength) of the hamstrings was 60% or less of the concentric strength of the quadriceps, there was a 77% chance of hamstring strain (Dauty *et al.*, 2003).

Developing eccentric strength will be covered in Chapter 12. The 'Nordic hamstring exercise' is strongly recommended.

Stretching During Warm-Up

Sports science generally indicates that static stretching during warm-ups will increase the chance of injury and will reduce an athlete's power. Stretching will be discussed in more detail in Chapter 8, but it must also be addressed now because static stretching during warm-up seems to be a major factor in causing hamstring strains. Research results vary because studies do not list exactly which exercises used were static, which were dynamic, and for how long the subjects stretched. However, the better designed studies indicate an increased injury potential from static stretching during the warm-up.

Why should this be? The major hypothesis concerns the elements which make the muscle contract. The actin in the sarcomeres that move up on the myosin through the action of crossbridges is weakened because the actin is pulled too far from the myosin so that there are not enough crossbridges left to make the unit shorten effectively. This might explain both the propensity for injury, by pulling them apart, and the loss of power, because there are not enough crossbridges connecting the two proteins to allow the sarcomere to contract fully. Another theory is that the connective tissue that holds the muscle cells together is stretched. This may weaken the whole muscle–tendon unit (*see* diagram on p. 30).

Some athletes, such as dancers, may strain their muscles while doing the stretch. Other athletes are less likely to do the extreme stretching that dancers do. Their injuries are more likely to occur during running or cutting. The data on dancers comes from a Swedish study (Askling *et al.*, 2002), which showed that 34% of the dancers studied had suffered an acute hamstring injury and another 17% had experienced a hamstring overuse injury during the previous ten years. Of all these injuries, 88% were suffered while doing slow stretching exercises. So obviously stretching the hamstring muscle–tendon tissues is not harmless to any athlete.

It seems that the longer players hold their stretches in their warm-ups the more likely they are to incur a hamstring strain. A study of the top four professional leagues in the UK found that 11% of all injuries were hamstring strains and that 14% of those were re-injuries (Dadebo *et al.*, 2004).

Recommendations

Muscle pulls often occur to players who:

- have done warm-up static stretching
- have a weak quadriceps-to-hamstring ratio (hamstrings should be at least 75% to 80% as strong as the quadriceps)

• stop and cut with only a small angle at the knee.

Players, especially girls, who tend to not get a sharp enough angle at the knee, should be trained in proper cutting and stopping techniques in which the knees are more sharply angled so that the muscles, rather than the ligaments, absorb more of the shock.

Dynamic stretching during the warm-up is essential (*see* Chapter 8 for more on warm-up and warm-up stretching).

The hamstrings must be strengthened so that they reach as close as 75–80% of the strength of the quadriceps as is possible. They should be strengthened both concentrically and eccentrically (*see* Chapter 12).

The hamstrings should be thoroughly warmed up through slow running progressing to sprinting. Since the effect of warm-up is nearly eliminated after ten minutes of inactivity or slow activity it would be wise for players, particularly older players, to do some short sprints, even when not necessary, during a match. Substitutes should also be warmed up before entering the match.

THE HIP AND TORSO

As regards the use of hips and torso, there may be differences between male and female players which affects their risk of injury. In a study of male and female collegiate soccer players who were tested on cutting moves to change direction while running (Pollard *et al.*, 2004), video analysis showed that females demonstrated significantly less peak hip abduction than did males; that is, the thighs of women players did not move as far from the midline of their bodies. However

it was concluded that male and female collegiate soccer players demonstrated similar hip and knee joint mechanics while performing cutting manoeuvres.

THE SHOULDER, ARM AND HANDS

Shoulder and arm injuries are most likely to occur from falls. The shoulder injury most commonly seen in soccer is a shoulder separation, a form of ligament sprain in the shoulder. Most require just protective padding, ice, and measures for pain control. Some more severe ligament tears may require surgery. Another less common injury is a shoulder dislocation, which may be partial or complete. A complete dislocation must be manipulated back into socket by a doctor.

Goalkeepers are especially at risk of these injuries. The frequent diving makes a keeper more likely to injure the shoulder and elbow. Catching and blocking balls may also cause injuries to the wrist and hand.

Recommendations

While all players may profit from the following suggestions they should be almost mandatory for goalkeepers. Doing shoulder strengthening exercises, such as flys (lateral raises), forward raises and bench presses will help to strengthen the shoulder joint (*see* Chapter 12).

Learning to fall without breaking the fall with the arm, or learning how to roll when falling would reduce the shoulder and arm injuries caused by falling. Players can be taught to dive flat out on to the grass without using their arms to break the fall. They can also learn to do shoulder rolls in which the weight is transferred from the back of the hand along the back of the arm then diagonally across the back.

SUMMARY

It is impossible to prevent all soccer injuries. Appropriate equipment is a must. Shin guards are mandatory. Goalkeepers should wear gloves to prevent hand injuries. Conditioning with both agility and endurance is needed. Strength and speed are also needed in soccer. Play it safe. When injuries occur, have the player evaluated by an athletic trainer or physician.

CHAPTER 8

Warm-Up

Warming up can be called 'getting up to speed' or readying the body for the task ahead. It starts in the dressing room, often with a routine of doing things in a certain order so that players can 'get in the groove'. Athletes from all sports employ these rituals, and tailor them to their needs. They can be fixed, and may hark back to a good win, a good goal, anything which had a good outcome.

Many players begin the process with music to help them concentrate; some will use rousing music or if a player suffers pre-match anxiety they may prefer calming or comforting music, such as a favourite from home. Most professional teams now have communal music, often the same for each game. This aids mental preparation, and may help recall triumphs. If the team loses, these rituals may change.

Once élite players get out onto the pitch or field, the physical side of warm-up starts. The mental side of the preparation can be interrupted at this time by fans and autograph hunters, and this is why, at this time, autographs are usually declined at the request of the coach or manager.

The physical warm-up usually consists of a slow jog to start, picking up speed gradually. This is all aerobic, and will increase the heart rate to about 50% of the maximum with a pulse of 90 to 120 beats per minute. Physiologically, the small blood vessels in the muscle bed (capillaries) open up and start to deliver oxygen and other nutrients. Simultaneously, the heart rate increases so that it can pump enough blood to the now exercising, and hence more demanding, muscles. After a short while, in well-trained players, a steady state will be reached where the blood (and oxygen) being pumped to the muscle is enough to keep them exercising without increasing greatly the heart rate, or rate of breathing. The player, whilst initially feeling slightly out of breath, now feels comfortable.

Next, there is a period of dynamic stretching. Stretching can be split into two types: passive and dynamic. In the past passive stretching, like toe touching, was thought to be the best at preventing injury. The theory was that if suppleness could be aided by stretching, and increasing the range of motion of that muscle group around a joint, then muscle and tendon injuries would be minimized, as they would not be stretched beyond their limit. However, it has been found recently that passive stretching does not reduce injuries, and may in fact increase them. Stretching also results in a reduction in the power output of that muscle.

Passive stretching has its place, not before exercise, but *after*, when the muscle and the connective tissue it lies in is slowly returned to the normal length. Passive stretching was always cited as good for stiffness that came on for the couple of days after exercise (delayed onset muscle soreness, DOMS), but even this has been shown not to be the case.

Dynamic stretching has, therefore, come to the fore in the pre-match warm-up. This encourages the neuro–muscular pathways to be alert, in preparation for the match. Dynamic stretching is done by taking the muscle–joint complex through a movement pattern that mimics what may happen in a game, rather like an orchestra warming up.

Finally comes a series of short sprints, which usually take the form of game simulation. This can be with a ball or just shadow play, sometimes using cones or markers. Then there is a period of free play, where players use the ball to pass to each other, again, often using rehearsal, both mental and physical. The coach may at this stage help some players with specific technique rehearsal.

Warm-up for goalkeepers is specific to their position. Although doing similar things, they will concentrate more on specific rehearsal than the outfield players. Most of the warm-up is used in shot stopping, diving and catching balls kicked in towards the goal. In general, goalkeepers have low aerobic capacities. They do not need to be aerobically fit, but they do need to have jumping and catching ability to go with quick reflexes.

THE NEGATIVE EFFECTS OF STATIC STRETCHING

Most coaches in previous years have been taught to warm-up their athletes by doing a number of stretches and some movement exercises such as running. The research indicates that, particularly for sports in which running is important, stretching can predispose players to injury, particularly to muscle and tendon injuries.

The reasons we have been given for stretching include:

- warming up the muscles and making them more ready to contract
- reducing the amount of DOMS, which is common, particularly in untrained or poorly trained exercisers
- reducing the chance for muscle injuries.

The research indicates that all three of these reasons are probably wrong for most people who exercise. A number of studies indicate that muscles function less well after stretching because the 'stiffness' required for maximal force is thereby reduced. DOMS does not seem to be reduced by stretching or massage. Muscle and connective tissue injuries are generally higher among those who stretch.

An analysis of all or most of the known studies in the area (Shrier, 1999) has shown that stretching alone generally does not prevent injuries. It either did not prevent injuries or it increased injuries. In further summarizing literature of basic physiology and anatomy it was found that:

- stretching does not increase the compliance (effective action) of a muscle during eccentric contractions; these lengthening contractions are most often associated with muscle and tendon injury
- stretching can produce damage at the cellular level of muscles and tendons
- stretching seems to mask muscular pain in humans, which is why stretching an injured muscle or tendon may make it feel better even though additional damage may be occurring

- stretching before an exercise will have no positive effect on a muscle which will not be required to elongate during the activity, such as jogging or walking; studies of joggers and slow runners indicate that stretching can cause injuries (O'Connor, 2003).

The first study that indicated that stretching might not be helpful was a survey done in 1983 (Kerner and D'Amico) of 500 runners. It found that those who warmed up had more injuries than those who did not (87% vs. 66%) and the frequency of injuries increased with the length of the warm-up. It is assumed that stretching was part of the warm-up but it was not specifically asked. A few years later a survey of 10K runners in the national championships found that those who stretched had more injuries (Jacobs and Berson, 1986). But it is not known whether those who stretched did so because they already had an injury and thought that the stretching would protect them from further injury. In a study of recreational distance runners over a whole year it was found that those who stretched sometimes had more injuries than those who always stretched or those who never stretched. But those who never stretched had fewer new injuries than those who stretched (Walter *et al.*, 1989).

Most muscle injuries occur in the normal range of motion, not in a lengthened state, so stretching will not reduce the causative factors. An Australian study (Pope *et al.*, 2000) of military recruits during twelve weeks of training, with half doing stretching exercises and half not, found that 'a typical muscle stretching protocol performed during pre-exercise warm-ups does not produce clinically meaningful reduc-

tions in risk of exercise-related injury in army recruits'.

Now that stretching is actually being investigated as a warm-up activity we have found a number of studies which show that it decreases one's power. The various studies show that stretching during warm-up decreases power by 4 to 8%. Why should this be so? Some, like Dr Arnold Nelson at Louisiana State University, believe that it is because the tendons are stretched so they become more slack. The contracting muscle must therefore take up the slack of the stretched tendon before it can tighten the tendon sufficiently to move the joint. Others believe that the problem lies in the sarcomere, the small muscle cell which holds the contractile elements. It is thought that the contractile elements, actin and myosin, are pulled further apart by the stretching so the muscle contraction must make up for that separation before the contraction can begin to be effective (AAHPERD, 2002). Still another possibility for the reduction in power is that when a person stretches, the number of neural impulses from the brain are decreased. It might therefore take longer to bring the number of neural impulses up to normal to begin more vigorous contractions. This is only a temporary phenomenon, but may be important if the player has suddenly to act early in a game, but does not have the power available when putting their 'foot on the gas'.

Some people stretch because they believe that it will reduce the soreness that can follow exercise. A Swedish study (Johansson *et al.*, 1999) investigated whether stretching would decrease DOMS in women doing eccentric exercise, the type of exercise most likely to increase muscle soreness. No advantages for stretching were found. The amount of soreness and tenderness was not reduced (*see also* Gullick, 1995; Rodenburg *et al*., 1994; High and Howley, 1989).

Increasing one's range of motion by stretching prior to exercise also does not seem to work (Cornelius and Hands, 1992). Since muscle strains are more likely to happen within the normal range of movement, stretching should not be a benefit if this is the reason for stretching.

Perhaps the most important results came from a British study of eighteen professional footballers, which looked at stretching and more soccer-specific skills (Little and Williams, 2004). They were tested with no stretching, static stretching and active stretching on the squat jump, 10m sprint (acceleration), flying 20m sprint (all-out speed) and 20m zig-zag sprint for agility. For the squat jump no stretching was best, dynamic stretching was second best, then static stretching. In the other tests dynamic stretching was best.

An interesting result came from a UK study of nearly a hundred rugby players, tested doing 20-yard sprints from standing starts. It found that the static stretching increased their times while those who actively stretched (while jogging) decreased their 20-yard times[4]. The differences represented about a yard difference between the static and the active stretchers in the 20-yard sprint.

Despite this negative commentary on static stretching, it should be mentioned that perhaps some people should stretch passively. One study found that when people did static stretching then were tested on a squat jump, about 40% jumped lower than they did when they did not stretch. About 50% had little change. But 10% jumped higher. A reason for this might be that they had very tight muscles. (The actin bodies were quite close to each other so that they were able to move only a little before the sarcomere had reached its maximum contraction. By stretching the actins further apart they had more potential to contract, see the drawing on p. 30 in Chapter 3.) If this study is representative of the general population of athletes, perhaps 10% of athletes could profit by static stretching. It is an area that has not yet been researched.

WARM-UP AND MUSCLE EFFICIENCY

There is no disagreement at this time about using sport-specific movements in the warm-up. Running, jumping, kicking and passing all seem to be effective in opening the blood supply to the muscles that will be used in the game or practice.

There is basic scientific evidence to suggest that active warm-up may be protective against muscle strain injury. Warming the muscles should be done by slowly doing sport-specific movements. In the case of soccer these are: jog, run, jump (as if heading), cut, then passing and kicking at goal.

A German study on the calf muscles (Rosenbaum and Hennig, 1995) measured muscle reflexes and force development after stretching, or running ten minutes, or with no prior warm-up. It indicated that the force development was about the same for the running warm-up and no warm-up and was

---

4   Those who did static stretches increased their times in the 20-yard sprint by 0.04 (passive static slow stretch) and 0.05 (active static stretch), while those who did dynamic stretches reduced their 20-yard time by 0.06 seconds (active dynamic stretch) and 0.03 (static dynamic stretch – dynamic movements done while standing).

considerably less (about 5% less) after stretching. There was, however, a great deal of difference between the fifty subjects in how each reacted to the various types of warm-up. This may indicate that some people need to be stretched in their warm-up, while most people do not. A Japanese study (Nosaka and Clarkson, 1997), using only five women as a part of a larger study, found that the warm-up reduced the amount of muscle damage caused by eccentric contractions.

Even a slight physical warm-up can increase the ability of the muscles to pick up oxygen through increased mitochondrial activity, according to a study at the University of Pennsylvania (Nioka et al., 1998). Even a somewhat relaxed movement pattern can help the muscles to bridge the gap from anaerobic to aerobic energy production.

WARM-UP AND ANAEROBIC CAPACITY INCREASE

Anaerobic energy is that produced without oxygen. In soccer it can be a quick burst of running or a keeper diving for the ball. An Australian study (involving full speed cycling for one minute) had one warm-up of four thirty-second maximum sprints and one of applying hot packs to the quadriceps muscles for an hour. Those who had actively warmed up had greater potential to use oxygen during the first thirty seconds of the test (O'Brien et al., 1997).

While admitting that there is little scientific support for the benefits of warm-up, athletes commonly warm-up prior to activity with the intention of improving performance and reducing the incidence of injuries. A Canadian study (Stewart and Sleivert, 1998), which compared a group not warming up with groups warming up at 60, 70 and 80% of their VO_2 max (the maximum amount of oxygen that an athlete can use in one minute), recommended a fifteen minute warm-up at 60 to 70% of the VO_2 max. The warm-up groups followed their aerobic warm-up with leg stretches. It was found that while ankle and hip extension ranges of movement were increased under all warm-up protocols, hip flexion increased only when the exercise warm-up was at 80% of maximum. The maximum anaerobic potentials were realized after the 70% VO_2 max warm-up.

WARM-UP AND INCREASED ENDURANCE

Warming up appears to improve endurance. A French study (Mandengue et al., 1996) used untrained young men exercising to exhaustion on a bicycle exerciser at 75% of their maximum heart rate. One trial was without a warm-up and one was with a fifteen minute warm-up (50% of maximum heart rate). The warm-up was found to allow better adjustment of the heat-regulating mechanisms of the body and the blood flow. It also increased the water loss during physical work. For most subjects, these adjustments allowed for improved endurance during the exercise.

RECOMMENDED WARM-UP

Based on research results it would seem that most people should not stretch statically. In fact probably no one should stretch because the stretching reduces the muscles' stiffness and their ability to contract to the maximum.

Heart rate and oxygen volume

The American College of Sports Medicine (ACSM) recommends using 220 heart beats per minute as a theoretical maximum. To find the maximum for a player, subtract his or her age from that 220. Aerobic exercise would be done at 60–90% of their maximum heart rate. So for a twenty year old it would be 220 – 20 = 200 (theoretical maximum); 60% of that would be a pulse rate of 120 and 90% would be a pulse rate of 180 beats per minute.

The VO_2 max (maximum volume of oxygen) is the major physiological measurement of aerobic capacity used by exercise physiologists. It determines the amount of oxygen that a body can use to develop energy while exercising.

The maximum amount of oxygen used (VO_2 max) is the number of millilitres (mL) of oxygen (O_2) per kilogram of body weight per minute. The approximate VO_2 max if working at 70% of one's maximum heart rate would be about 85. A 90% of maximum heart rate would be about an 88 VO_2 max. The highest VO_2 max ever recorded was in a Norwegian cross country skier. It was 96.

It also seems to set them up for more chance of injury during eccentric contractions, which occur in most running and jumping activities. The exception would be for those with overly tight muscles (contractures) whose efficiency will be increased by reducing the excessive tightness. On the other hand, dynamic, sport-specific stretching should be a part of the warm-up.

The research tells us that about fifteen minutes of exercise at about 60–70% of the athlete's VO_2 max should be effective. Certainly the warm-up in soccer will have

to include some maximal efforts, such as jumping, sprinting and kicking.

Contrary to popular belief, there is little, if any, evidence that warm-up prevents or reduces the risk of injury (Maughan and Shirreffs, 2004). It does, however, get the body functioning more efficiently if the weather is cold. There is also the possible psychological effect of focusing on the task at hand. The amount of warm-up depends on how much time it takes to get the heart beating faster (about 60–70% of one's maximum heart rate) and to get blood flowing to the muscles, including the muscles used in breathing.

It does not take long to ready the body to function effectively in warmer climates. In hot climates one should not warm-up the body too much because performance can be decreased and fatigue can set in earlier. This is consistent with the emerging evidence that a marked rise in body temperature – especially in brain temperature – is a major factor in causing fatigue during prolonged exercise in the heat (Nybo et al., 2002). In fact in hot weather, once the blood is flowing, it may be wise to cool the body with cold towels, cold showers, colder wet clothing and electric fans in order to keep the brain, blood and muscles at a more optimal operating temperature. This would be particularly desirable at halftime.

RECOMMENDED COOL-DOWN

After the practice or game, stretching may not hurt, but any excessive stretching may set up the muscle fibres for injury during the next practice. There is no evidence that post-exercise stretching will increase flexibility or reduce DOMS, yet these were the reasons often given for stretching after the practice or game. Stretching for an increased range of motion should have been done very early in the sporting season, in fact immediately after the last season.

Some post-exercise jogging may assist in reducing the blood pooling in the muscles, but if bruises, strains or sprains were incurred in the practice or game the extra work might increase the blood flow to the injury and increase the swelling when it should have been treated with ice or cold to reduce any potential swelling.

There have been few studies on the effects of cool-down. A study in Japan (Koyama *et al.*, 2000) of older cardiac patients (aged 50–70) found that after a maximal cardiac exercise, those who used a cool-down period rather than just resting had a more efficient return to normal in terms of breathing. The resting group hyperventilated and had a more uneven return to the resting state. A 1993 Dutch study (van Mechelen *et al.*) used over 300 runners; half of them were given information on preventing running injuries, including how to warm-up, stretch and cool-down. A diary was kept for sixteen weeks by each runner noting what was done and how many injuries occurred. Those who received the information had 5.5 injuries per thousand hours of running. Those who did not get the information had 4.9 injuries per thousand hours of running. The conclusion of the study was that the information was the first step in preventing injuries but perhaps the study's assumption that warm-up, stretching and cool-down will prevent injuries is wrong, or at least wrong for most runners.

CHAPTER 9
Nutrition

An athlete cannot be in top condition without having sufficient amounts of the essential nutrients. A basic understanding of nutrition is essential to healthy living, and in athletes, to reaching full playing potential. This chapter deals with general nutrition and will also point out some of the relationships between food and exercise.

Very few people consume even the minimum amounts of each of the necessary nutrients: protein, fat, carbohydrates, vitamins, minerals and the essential non-nutrient, water. The first three (protein, fat and carbohydrates) bring with them the energy required for practice and play.

The 'calorie' used in counting food energy is really a Kilocalorie (Kc), one thousand times larger than the calorie used as a measurement of heat in chemistry. In one Kilocalorie there is enough energy to heat 1kg of water 1 degree Celsius (2.2 pounds 1.8 degrees Fahrenheit), or to lift 3,000 pounds of weight one foot high. So those calories listed on food packaging pack a lot of energy.

Most people need about 17Kc per pound of body weight per day in order to keep themselves functioning in their normal daily activities. Most athletes, particularly the endurance athletes, need much more. Playing soccer uses about another 4Kc per pound per hour.

THE MAJOR NUTRIENTS

Protein

Protein is composed of amino acids, of which there are twenty-two that are important for humans. Amino acids are made up of carbon, hydrogen, oxygen and nitrogen. While both fats and carbohydrates contain the first three elements, nitrogen is found only in protein. Protein is essential for building the cells that compose nearly every part of the body – the brain, heart, organs, skin, muscles and even the blood.

There are four calories in one gram of protein. Adults require 0.75g of protein per kilogram of body weight per day. This translates into one-third of a gram of protein per pound. So, an easy estimate for protein requirements in grams per day would be to divide the body weight by three. For instance, an athlete weighing 150 pounds needs about 50 grams of protein per day. Strength athletes have been found to need 1.2–1.7g of protein per kilogram of body weight. Some researchers have studied intakes as high as 2.4g per day. It seems that 1.6 grams per day for soccer players is more than sufficient. To put it simply, to take 12–15% of daily calories in protein provides all that is needed. Excess protein consumption (above the body's requirement) will be broken down and the calories will either be burned off or stored as fat.

Amino acids

To make and repair any body organ, including muscle, requires all of the necessary amino acids. Some of them your body can manufacture, while others you must get from your food. Those amino acids that you must get from your food are called the essential amino acids, while those that you can make are known as the non-essential amino acids.

Amino acids cannot be stored in the body. Therefore, people need to consume their minimum amounts of protein every day. If adequate protein is not consumed, the body immediately begins to break down tissue (usually beginning with muscle tissue) to release the essential amino acids. If even one essential amino acid is lacking, the others are not able to work to their full capacities. For example, if methionine (the most commonly lacking amino acid) is present at 60% of the minimum requirement, the other seven essential amino acids are limited to near 60% of their potential. When they are not used, amino acids are deaminated and excreted as urea in the urine.

Animal products (fish, poultry and meat) and animal by-products (milk, milk products and eggs) are rich in readily usable protein. These foods are called complete protein sources.

Incomplete protein sources are any other food sources that provide protein but not high levels of all of the essential amino acids. Some examples of incomplete proteins include beans, peas and nuts. These food sources must be combined with other food sources that have the missing essential amino acids so

that protein can be made in the body. Some examples of complementary foods are rice with beans, or peanut butter on wholewheat bread. The highest rated proteins, according to their amino acid content, are:

- egg whites (94–98% complete)
- non-fat milk (88–92%)
- fish (about 88%)
- chicken and other fowl (about 85%)
- organ meats (82%)
- beef steak (78%)
- soya (72%)
- wholegrain wheat (65%)
- beans (58%)
- peanuts (54%).

Protein supplements

Weight trainers, in particular among athletes, are keen on protein supplements, but they may not be good value because they usually fall far short of an effective balance of the essential amino acids. While six of the essential amino acids are usually present in good quantities in these supplements, methionine and tryptophan are usually found in lesser amounts, and they are the most commonly lacking. Since 6mg per pound of methionine (13mg per kg) and 1.6g of tryptophan (3.5g per kg) per day are the recommended daily allowances, it is important to check how much of these are actually contained in a supplement. This is especially important in a diet lacking in either one or both of these amino acids and which relies primarily on the supplement for most or all of its protein needs. A better and cheaper source of protein for one needing a supplement would be powdered milk. A diet deficient in protein might also be improved with egg whites (or egg substitutes), milk, fish or chicken. It may prove less expensive and more nutritious.

Fats

Fat is made of carbon, hydrogen and oxygen. There are nine calories in a gram of fat. In the body, fat is used to develop the myelin sheath that surrounds the nerves. It also aids in the absorption of vitamins A, D, E, and K, which are fat soluble. It serves as a protective layer around our vital organs, and is a good insulator against the cold. It is also a highly concentrated energy source. Its most redeeming quality is that it adds flavour and juiciness to food.

Just as protein is broken down into different kinds of nitrogen compounds called amino acids, there are also different kinds of fats. There are three major kinds of fats (fatty acids): saturated fats, monounsaturated fats, and polyunsaturated fats. A more newly recognized fat is called a trans-fatty acid, which occurs when an unsaturated fat is converted to a harder saturated-like fat in foods. This occurs when oils, such as corn and safflower oil, are hardened to make margarines.

There is evidence of hardened arteries even in children in England and America, so if players want to live longer they should be concerned with the amount and types of fat they consume.

Saturated fats

These fats are 'saturated' with hydrogen atoms. They are generally solid at room temperature and are most likely found in animal fats, egg yolks and whole milk products. Since these are the fats that are primarily responsible for raising blood cholesterol level and hardening the arteries, they should be kept to a minimum in the diet.

Monounsaturated fats

Also called oleic fatty acids, these are liquid at room temperature and are found in great amounts in olive, peanut, and rapeseed (canola) oils. Dietary monounsaturated fats have been shown to have the greatest effect on the reduction of cholesterols, particularly the most harmful low-density lipoproteins (LDLs), thereby contributing a positive effect on atherosclerosis.

Polyunsaturated fats

These linoleic fatty acids are also liquid at room temperature and are found in the highest proportions in vegetable sources. Safflower, corn and linseed oils are good sources of this type of fat. Polyunsaturated fatty acids of the omega-3 type, found primarily in fatty fish (especially salmon, trout, mackerel and herring) may also contribute to the prevention of atherosclerosis.

Trans-fatty acids

These are particularly harmful fats that are made commercially when hydrogen atoms are added to unsaturated fats to make them hard at room temperature. The words 'partially hydrogenated vegetable oils' on a food label show that the product contains these harmful fats. The US government is now requiring the reduction and eventually the elimination of these fats, which are found commonly in margarines, biscuits and crackers.

Carbohydrates

Carbohydrates are made from carbon, hydrogen, and oxygen, as are fats, but are generally a simpler type of molecule. There are four calories in a gram of carbohydrate. If not utilized immediately for energy as sugar (glucose), they are either stored in the body as glycogen (the stored form of glucose) or synthesized into fat and stored. Some carbohydrates cannot be broken down by the body's digestive processes. These are called fibres.

Of the digestible carbohydrates, there are two categories: simple and complex. Simple carbohydrates are the most readily usable energy source for the body and include such things as sugar, honey, and fruit. Complex carbohydrates are the starches. Complex 'carbs' also break down into sugar for energy, but their breakdown is slower than with simple ones. Also, complex carbohydrates bring with them various vitamins, minerals and fibres.

Since the energy used in both strength and power conditioning and on the field should come from sugars (glucose, glycogen, etc.), which are stored in the body, soccer players must be conscious of consuming plenty of carbohydrates – but not enough to put on body fat.

Water

Water is called the essential non-nutrient because it brings with it no nutritional value and yet, without it, we would die. Water makes up approximately 60% of the adult body. It is used to cool the body through perspiration, to carry nutrients to the cells

Checklist for reading a food label

1 Read the ingredients. Generally the ingredients are listed in order, according to the proportions used in the product. Those concerned with the amount and types of fats in the product should look for: whole eggs or egg yolks, cream or whole milk, butter or other animal fats, margarine or hydrogenated vegetable fats (sometimes listed as partially hardened fats), palm kernel oil or coconut oil. These are primarily saturated fats. If the percentage of saturated fat is 12% or more, it is too high.

2 Look at the nutritional analysis.

- How many calories (Kcal) are there per serving?
- What is the percentage of total fat? Multiply the number of grams of fat by 9 then divide that number into the total calories. If that number is less than 10% it is acceptable. The maximum recommended is 30%.
- What is the proportion of saturated fat? If the label breaks down the fats into saturated, mono-unsaturated and poly-unsaturated fats, make certain that the saturated fats are less than a third of total fats (lower is better).
- Are there hydrogenated vegetable fats? These contain trans-fats, which act similarly to saturated fats but will be listed as unsaturated fats, so you must refer back to the ingredients list to check for hydrogenated vegetable fats or partially hardened fats.
- Is there any fibre? Any fibre is good, more than 4g per 100g is excellent.
- Are vitamins listed? Check the percentage of the recommended daily allowance (RDA). If the less common vitamins, such as B6, B12 and E are included in the list, that is good.

and waste products away from them, to help cushion our vital organs, and is a principle ingredient in all body fluids.

The body has about 18 square feet (1.6sq. m) of skin that contains about 2 million sweat glands. On a comfortable day, a person will perspire about a half pint of water. A soccer player exercising on a severely hot day may lose as much as 8–15 pints (4–8L) of water. This needs to be replaced or severe dehydration can result.

Vitamins

Vitamins are organic compounds that are essential in small amounts for the growth and development of animals and humans. They act as enzymes (catalysts), which facilitate many of bodily processes. Although there is some controversy as to the importance of consuming excess vitamins, it is acknowledged that we need a minimum amount of vitamins for proper functioning. Now that the destructive impact of free oxygen radicals (due largely to exercise and air pollution) has been established, it is generally recommended that certain vitamins, such as C, E and beta carotene, be included in the daily intake of these nutrients at levels higher than those formerly recommended. (*See* table on p. 88.)

Some vitamins are soluble only in water; others need fat to be absorbed by the body.

The water-soluble vitamins

Vitamin B complex and vitamin C are water-soluble and more fragile than the fat-soluble vitamins. This is because they are more easily destroyed by the heat of cooking and, if boiled, they lose a little of their potency into the water. Since they are not stored by the body, they should be included in the daily diet.

Vitamins B1 and B3 help to break down sugars so that they can be used by the muscles. B2 helps to break down fats that are used for energy. B6 helps to break down proteins into amino acids. B12 is used to develop the blood cells that carry oxygen to the muscles. Vitamin C is essential in the production of collagen, the protein substance that is the mainstay of the body's connective tissues, including tendons, ligaments and other body tissues, such as bones, teeth and skin. It also is important for healing wounds and in developing the body's immune defence which fights off infection. In addition it helps the body to use iron and it assists in the creation of the thyroid hormone thyroxin.

The fat-soluble vitamins

Vitamins A, D, E and K need oils in the intestines to be absorbed by the body. They are more stable than the water-soluble vitamins and are not destroyed by normal cooking methods. Vitamin A helps eyesight, D helps to build strong bones, E is important in heart health and K helps in blood clotting.

Minerals

Minerals are usually structural components of the body, but they sometimes participate in certain body processes. (*See* table on p. 92.) Iron is essential for making the haemoglobin that carries the oxygen in the red blood cells. Magnesium helps to develop energy and is important in the contraction of the heart and muscle fibres. Calcium builds strong bones and is also essential in the blood and in the contraction of muscles. Insufficient calcium can be a cause of muscle cramps. Potassium is essential for cell growth, which can cause muscle weakness. It also aids in keeping the blood's chemical balance stable during exercise.

Sodium helps to maintain the body's water balance. Since it is the major mineral ingredient in sweat it occasionally needs to be increased in very hot weather or when the athlete perspires too much. A lack of sodium or calcium can contribute to cramping.

Trace minerals

These are the minerals that are found in very small amounts. Copper helps in the production of red blood cells. It also helps in the metabolism of glucose, with the release of energy, in the formation of fats in the nerve walls, and of connective tissues. Manganese is used in fat and carbohydrate metabolism and aids in muscle function. Zinc is used in carbohydrate metabolism and it aids in wound healing. Chromium helps to regulate blood sugar and to metabolize fats and carbohydrates. It is also an antioxidant.

Supplementation with Vitamins and Minerals

Athletes commonly supplement their nutritional needs with vitamin or mineral pills. It is important only to use supplements that are actually needed, and such needs vary according to individuals. Most people will probably profit from taking a complete multivitamin and mineral supplement. Most women will want iron as one of the minerals; most men do not need extra iron. Menstruating women need 18mg a day of iron while men require only 10mg. Those on a weight-reducing diet may well need a multivitamin and mineral supplement as their intake is likely to be imbalanced.

America's most famous fitness guru, Dr Ken Cooper, who started the aerobics revolution, believes we should supplement our diets with certain vitamins and minerals, particularly the antioxidants. Although many believe that all the necessary vitamins and minerals can be acquired from our diet, Cooper says that it cannot really be done. In fact we need more of some nutrients than we could possibly take in through a normal diet. He recommends:

- 25,000 units of beta carotene
- 1,000mg of vitamin C
- 400mg of vitamin E (specifically d-alpha tocopherol, the natural form of vitamin E)
- 400μg of folacin
- some co-enzyme Q10.

His message is that 'You can age fast or age slow – it's up to you.'

Endurance athletes benefit from higher doses of antioxidants. Cooper suggests that anyone exercising more than five hours weekly should double the recommended dosage to combat excess free radical by-products. There are a number of antioxidants but the major ones are beta carotene, selenium and vitamins C and E.

The only dangers in taking high doses of vitamins seem to be with vitamin A if it is consumed in its animal form. Beta carotene, the vegetable precursor to vitamin A, seems to be no problem. Doses of vitamin E of over 400 units may be a problem for some.

NUTRITION AND RECOVERY

It seems obvious that eating the right food at the right time is the only way to get the best out of a player. There is debate about the best time to eat before a game, but 3–3½ hours is the norm. The meal should be a mixture of simple and complex carbohydrates, with protein in the way of non-fatty meat such as chicken, or fish.

After playing, there should always be low fat foods available for players. The body is depleted of carbohydrate, and while it takes about twenty-four hours to become replete again, absorption and storage is most efficient in the first four hours. The first hour is the most efficient in absorbing the needed carbohydrates. If there are foods available in the dressing room, players will take these on board, and by the next training session will be fully carbohydrate loaded.

In tournaments, where games and training come thick and fast, this can make the difference between winning and losing. If a player has no carbohydrate, he or she will not be able to keep up, and this could cost the team the game. After the initial snack in the dressing room, the player should eat a balanced meal within four hours.

Hydration

Hydration is just as important. Track and field athletes, especially long distance runners, have always known the benefits of retaining hydration, but it is easier to take on fluid in an individual sport than in a team sport where the breaks are few. If a player is out of position whilst getting a drink and the opposition scores, this can be disconcerting to all, to say the least.

Vitamin	Solubility	RDA	Functions	Deficiencies and excesses	Sources
A	Fat soluble stored in body	Men: 5,000 units (RE retinal equiva-lents) Women: 4,000 units (800 RE) Toxic level: 10,000 to 50,000 units (2,000 to 10,000 RE) (if all from animal sources)	1. Formation of body tissue 2. Development of mucous secretions in nose, mouth digestive tract, organs (which show bacterial entry) 3. Development of visual purple in the retina of the eye, which allows one to see in the dark 4. Produces the enamel-producing cells of the teeth 5. Assists normal growth 6. Estrogen synthesis 7. Sperm production	Deficiencies can cause night blindness, damaged intestinal tract, damaged reproductive tract, scaly skin, poor bones, dry mucous membranes, and in children, poor enamel in the teeth. Toxic symptoms (of Retinol): may mimic brain tumour (increased pressure inside the skull), weight loss, irritability, loss of appetite, severe headaches, vomiting, itching, menstrual irregularities, diarrhoea, fatigue, skin lesions, bone and joint pains, loss of hair, liver and spleen enlargement, and insomnia. In children, overdose can stunt growth.	Butter and margarine, whole milk, liver, fish, fortified non-fat milk, fish-liver oils, egg yolk.
Beta-carotene		As antioxidant 25,000 to 50,000 units (15 to 30mg)	1. Precursor to vitamin A 2. Antioxidant – Reduces cancer risk – Reduces heart disease	Deficiency: increased free oxygen radical activity. Excess: may yellow the skin	Carrots, broccoli, dark green or orange fruits or vegetables.
B1 (thiamin)	Water soluble	1.5mg (men) 1.2mg (women)	1. Metabolizes carbohydrates 2. Resulting glucose (sugar) nourishes muscles and nerves 3. Aids nerve functioning	Deficiencies can cause: mental depression, moodiness, quarrelsomeness and uncooperativeness, fatigue, irritability, lack of appetite, muscle cramps, constipation, nerve pains (due to degeneration of myelin sheath which covers the nerve), weakness and feeling	Liver, pork, yeast, organ meats, whole grains, bread, wheat germ, peanuts, milk, eggs, soya beans.

Vitamin	Solubility	RDA	Functions	Deficiencies and excesses	Sources
B1 (thiamin) *continued*				of heaviness in the legs, beri-beri (a disease in which the muscles atrophy and become paralysed)	
B2 (riboflavin)	Water soluble	1.8mg (men) 1.4mg (women)	1. Effects rate of growth and metabolic rate since it is necessary for the cell's use of protein, fat, and carbohydrate 2. Growth 3. Adrenal cortex activity 4. Red blood cells formation	Deficiencies can cause: burning and itching eyes, blurred and dim vision, eyes sensitive to light, inflammation of the lips and tongue, lesions at the edges of the mouth, digestive disturbances, greasy, scaly skin, personality problems	Eggs, liver and other organs, yeast, milk, whole grains, bread, wheat germ, green leafy vegetables
B3 (niacin or nicotinic acid)	Water soluble Limited storage in body	20mg (men) 15mg (women)	1. Similar to riboflavin in metabolizing foods (especially sugars) 2. Maintain normal skin conditions 3. Aids in functioning of the gastro-intestinal tract	Deficiencies can cause: dermatitis (red, tender skin, becoming scaly and ulcerated), fatigue, sore mouth (tongue), diarrhoea, vomiting, nervous disturbances, mental depression, anorexia, weight loss, headache, backache, mental confusion, irritability, hallucinations, delusion of persecution, pellagra. Large doses can be toxic because it dilates blood vessels. Can cause skin flushing, dizziness, head throbbing, also dryness of skin, itching, brown skin pigmentation, decreased glucose (sugar) tolerance and perhaps a rise in uric acid in the blood	Yeast, liver, wheat, bran, peanuts, beans
Pantothenic acid	Water soluble Little storage in body	4–7mg	1. Carbohydrate, fat and protein metabolism 2. Synthesis of cholesterol and steroid hormones 3. Aids the functioning of the adrenal cortex 4. Aids in choline metabolism	Almost never deficient in human diets. Various animal studies have shown different results from deficiency: rough skin, diarrhoea, anaemia, possible coma, convulsions, hair loss, and many other symptoms. But they have not been shown in humans	Liver, organ meats, yeast, wheat bran, legumes, cereals

Vitamin	Solubility	RDA	Functions	Deficiencies and excesses	Sources
Biotin	Water soluble	0–3mg	Metabolism of amino acids, fatty acids and carbohydrates	Deficiencies are extremely rare. Raw egg whites, which combine with the biotin in the intestines and make it unavailable and some antibiotics (which kill the biotin-producing organization in the intestines) could cause a deficiency. Deficiency would be marked by: dry, scaly skin, grey pallor (skin colour), slight anaemia, muscular pains, weakness, depression and loss of appetite	Manufactured in the intestines. Also found in: liver, yeast, kidney, egg yolks
B6 (pyridoxine)	Water soluble	2.0mg (men) 2.0mg (women)	1. Catalyst in protein, fat, and carbohydrate metabolism. High protein diet increases the need for B6 2. Converts tryptophan to niacin 3. Assists in nervous system 4. Antibody production	Anaemia, dizziness, nausea, vomiting, irritability, confusion, kidney stones, skin and mucous membrane problems. In infants: irritability, muscle twitching, convulsions. Excesses – impaired sensation in limbs. Unsteady gait	Usually not necessary to supplement. Wheatgerm, kidney, liver, ham, organ meats, legumes, peanuts
Folic acid (folacin)		0.2–0.4mg	1. Aids in maturation of red and white blood cells 2. May assist in the synthesis of nucleic acids 3. DNA synthesis	Blood disorders, anaemia, diarrhoea. Deficiencies most likely to occur during pregnancy and lactation	Yeast, liver, egg yolk, green leafy vegetables
B12	Water soluble, stored in the body	60mg (men and women)	1. Controls blood forming defects and nerve involvement in pernicious anaemia 2. Involved in protein, fat, carbohydrates, nucleic acid and folic acid metabolism 3. Necessary to the normal functioning of cells, especially in the bone marrow, nervous system and intestinal tract	Sore tongue, amenorrhoea, signs of degeneration of the spinal cord, anaemia, heart, and stomach trouble, headache, and fatigue	Liver, organ meats, oysters, salmon, eggs, beef, milk

Vitamin	Solubility	RDA	Functions	Deficiencies and excesses	Sources
C (ascorbic acid)	Water soluble. Little body storage	60mg; 10mg per day prevents scurvy Recommended as antioxidant: 1–1.5g	1. Forms collagen intracellular cement which strengthens cell walls (especially the small blood vessels and capillaries), tooth dentine, cartilage, bones and connective tissue 2. Aids in the absorption of iron 3. Aids in formation of red blood cells in the bone marrow 4. Aids in the metabolism of some amino acids (phenylalanine and tyrosine) 5. May be involved in the synthesis of steroid hormones from cholesterol 6. Any body stress may deplete the vitamin C in the tissues which may increase shock, or bacterial infections 7. Antioxidant	Scurvy results from low vitamin C intake. Minor symptoms of vitamin C deficiency could be: subcutaneous haemorrhages (bleeding below the skin), bleeding from gums, swollen gums. Excess of vitamin C can result in kidney stones and diarrhoea, destruction of B12, acidosis	Citrus, fresh fruits, berries, broccoli, tomatoes, green leafy vegetables, baked potatoes, turnips
D	Stored in liver Fat soluble	400 units (10mcgm) Toxic level: 1,000 to 1,500 units (25 to 38mcgm)	1. Assists in the development of bone and teeth by aiding calcium to harden 2. Facilitates the absorption of calcium and phosphorus, lack of which can cause muscular cramping. 3. Neuromuscular activity	Deficiencies: rickets (children), osteomalacia (women who have had frequent pregnancies and poor diets). Teeth may be more susceptible to caries (cavities). Cramping in muscles if there is a low level of calcium or phosphorus in the blood. Soft bones, bowed legs, poor posture. Toxic symptoms: fatigue, weight loss, nausea, vomiting, weakness, headache, kidney damage, kidney stones, hardening of the soft tissue of the heart, blood vessels, lungs, stomach and kidneys. Increase cholesterol level of	Exposure to ultraviolet light (sunshine) can give minimum daily requirements by changing one type of cholesterol to vitamin D. Milk, fish-liver oils, egg yolk, butter, whole milk. Non-fat milk (with D) Margarines (with D added)

Vitamin	Solubility	RDA	Functions	Deficiencies and excesses	Sources
D *continued*				blood. Makes bones more fragile. High levels in developing foetuses and young children may cause mental retardation or blood vessel retardation or blood vessel malformation (especially a blockage in the aorta – the major artery from the heart)	
E (tocopherol)	Fat soluble not stored in body	10 units 10mg TE (tocopherol equivalents) As an antioxidant: 400 units (TE) 600 units (if over 50 years, 2,500 if heavy exerciser)	1. It is thought to stabilize membranes 2. May be helpful in stabilizing Vitamin A 3. May be necessary in diets high in polyunsaturated fats 4. Aids in synthesizing red blood cells 5. Antioxidant	No known deficiency symptoms in human adults. Some premature infants apparently do not immediately develop the ability to absorb the vitamin	Synthesized in the intestines. Alpha tocopherol D Alpha tocopherol E better than mixed tocopherol E. Human milk (cow's milk poor), margarine, oil salad dressing, cereal germ, green leafy vegetables
K	Fat soluble	Men: 80mcgm. Women 63mcgm	Helps in the production of prothrombin (blood clotting agent)	Antibiotics taken orally (which could kill the synthesizing bacteria) or diarrhoea (which could flush out the bacteria) could possibly cause a deficiency. Newborn infants, especially premature babies, often suffer from a deficiency. This may cause excessive bleeding. Toxic symptoms in infants: jaundice, mild anaemia	Synthesized by intestinal bacteria. Green leafy vegetables, cabbage, cauliflower. Smaller amounts in: tomatoes, egg yolk and whole milk

Minerals	Solubility	RDA	Functions	Deficiencies and excesses	Sources
Calcium		1,200mg	Development of strong bones and teeth. Helps muscles contract and relax normally, utilization of iron. Normal blood clotting. Maintenance of body neutrality. Normal action of heart muscle	Rickets, porous bones, bowed legs, stunted growth, slow clotting of blood, poor tooth formation, tetany	Milk, cheese, mustard, turnip, green clams, oyster, broccoli, cauliflower, cabbage, molasses, nuts. Small amount in egg, carrot, celery, orange, grapefruit, figs, and bread made with milk

Mineral	Solubility	RDA	Functions	Deficiencies and excesses	Sources
Fluorine		1.5–4mg	Resistance to dental caries. Deposition of bone calcium. May be involved in iron absorption	Deficiencies: weak teeth and bones, anaemia, impaired growth. At levels of 1 5 to 4 parts per million teeth will be strong, but may be mottled. At levels over 6ppm teeth and bones may be deformed	Water supply containing 1ppm. Small amounts in many foods
Iodine		0.15mg	Constituent of thyroxin which is a regulator of metabolism. Synthesis of vitamin A	Enlarged thyroid gland. Low metabolic rate, stunted growth, retarded mental growth	Iodized salt sea foods, food gown in non-goitrous regions
Iron		10 mg (men) 15 mg (women)	Constituent of haemoglobin, which carries oxygen to the tissues. Collagen synthesis, antibody production	Nutritional anaemia, pallor, weight loss, fatigue, weakness, retarded growth	Red meats, especially liver, green vegetables, yellow fruits, prunes, raisins, legumes, whole grain and enriched cereals molasses, egg yolk, potatoes, oysters
Magnesium		350–400mg (men) 280–300mg (women)	Activates various enzymes. Assists in breakdown of phosphate and glucose necessary for muscle contractions. Regulates body temperature. Assist in synthesizing protein. Tooth enamel stability	Failure to grow, pallor, weakness, irritability of nerves and muscles, irregular heartbeat, heart and kidney damage, convulsions and seizures, delirium, depressions	Soya flour, whole wheat, oatmeal, peas, brown rice, whole corn, beans, nuts, soybeans, spinach, clams
Phosphorus		800–1,200mg (men & women)	Development of bones and teeth. Multiplication of cells. Activation of some enzymes and vitamins. Maintenance of body neutrality. Participates in carbohydrate metabolism. ADP/ATP synthesis acid/base balance. DNA/RNA synthesis	Rickets, porous bones, bowed legs, stunted growth, poor tooth formation. Excesses of phosphorus may have same effect on the bones as deficient calcium (osteoporosis porous bones)	Milk, cheese, meat, egg yolk, fish, nuts, whole grain cereals, legumes, soya flour, whole wheat, oatmeal, peas, brown rice, whole corn, beans
Potassium		2.5g	Acid-base balance. Carbohydrate metabolism.	Apathy, muscular weakness, poor gastro-intestinal tone, respiratory	Soya beans, cantaloupe, sweet potatoes, avocado, raisins,

Mineral	Solubility	RDA	Functions	Deficiencies and excesses	Sources
Potassium *continued*			Conduction of nerve impulses. Contraction of muscle fibres. May assist in lowering blood pressure (if consumed in equal proportions as sodium)	muscle failure, tachycardia (irregular heartbeat), cardiac arrest (heart stops beating)	banana, halibut, sole, baked beans, molasses, ham, mushroom, beef, white potatoes, tomatoes, kale, radishes, prune juice, nuts and seeds, wheat germ, green leafy vegetables, cocoa, vegetable juices, cream of tartar, prunes, figs, apricots, oranges, grapefruit
Selenium		70mcgm men 55mcgm women As an antioxidant up to 100 for heavy exercisers	Antioxidant – may reduce risk of stomach and oesophageal cancers	Toxic level: nausea, hair loss, diarrhoea, irritability	Organ meats, meats, milk, fruits (depends on the amount of selenium in the soil)
Sodium		1–2g (⅛ to ½ teaspoon)	Constraint of extra-cellular fluid. Maintenance of body neutrality. Osmotic pressure. Muscle and nerve irritability. Acid/base balance	Muscle cramps, weakness, headache, nausea, anorexia, vascular collapse. Excess may raise blood pressure	Sodium chloride (table salt), sodium bicarbonate (baking soda), monosodium glutamate. The greatest portion of sodium is provided by table salt and salt used in cooking. Foods high in sodium include: dried beef, ham, canned corned beef, bacon, wheat breads, salted crackers, flaked breakfast cereals, olives, cheese, butter, margarine, sausage, dried fish, canned vegetables, shellfish and salt water fish, raw celery, egg white
Zinc		15mg men 12mg women	Metabolism, formation of nucleic acid. Enzyme formation. Collagen production, fetal development, enhanced appetite and taste	Impaired growth, sexual development, skin problems	Beef, chicken, fish, beans, whole wheat, cashew nuts

RDA = Recommended (minimum) Daily Allowance

CHAPTER 10

Environmental Concerns: Heat, Hydration and Air Pollution

HEAT

Excess heat not only negatively affects an athlete's performance but it can also be a source of serious health problems. As the outside temperature increases it becomes harder to rid the body of the heat that exercise produces. For example, if exercising at 37°F (3°C) the body is 20% more effective in eliminating body heat than at 67°F (20°C) and 150% more effective than at 104°F (40°C). It is not uncommon for the body to reach a temperature of 104–106°F (40–41°C) when exercising. But normal resting body temperature is 98.6°F (37°C). The high heat makes it difficult, or impossible, for the perspiration to evaporate so the body cannot effectively be cooled. This increases fatigue and decreases performance.

The heat generated in the muscles is released by:

- conduction, from the warmer muscles to the cooler skin
- convection, from the heat loss from the skin to the air, and
- evaporation, of the perspiration being vaporized.

Conduction

Conduction occurs through the body's liquids, such as the blood, absorbing the heat created by the contraction of the muscles and moving it to the cooler skin. Water can absorb many thousands times more heat than can the air, so it is an excellent conductor of heat from the muscles.

Convection

Convection occurs when the heat near the skin is absorbed into the atmosphere. For a swimmer in a cool pool, effective convection is very easy. For the runner it is more difficult. Convection is aided by a lower air temperature and by wind. A 4mph (6km/h) wind is twice as effective in cooling as a 1mph (1.6km/h) wind.

Evaporation

This is the most effective method for cooling the body that is exercising in the air. Each litre of sweat that evaporates takes with it 580Kc. This is enough heat to raise the temperature of 10L of water by 58°C (21 pints of water by 105°F). As the skin is cooled by evaporation of the sweat, it is able to take more heat from the blood and thereby cool the blood so that it can pick up more heat from the muscles. Humidity is the most important factor regulating the evaporation of sweat.

High humidity reduces the ability of perspiration to evaporate. It is the evaporation of sweat that produces the cooling effect as perspiration changes from liquid to gas. This amounts to a cooling effect of over a half a kilocalorie per gram of perspiration evaporated. Exercising in a rubber suit has similar effects to high humidity because the water cannot evaporate – so it is not recommended.

Wind has the opposite effect. It affects the body temperature by cooling it faster than the registered temperature would warrant. We have all heard of the wind chill factor present on colder days. The wind makes the body experience more cold than would be expected by the actual temperature. But even on warmer days the wind will evaporate perspiration and cool the body faster than might otherwise be expected. This may increase the need for fluids in order to continue the production of sweat.

Fluid Replacement

The hyperthermia (high temperature) developed during exercise, particularly when sweat cannot evaporate, is a major cause of fatigue. This is particularly true when the body has lost 2% of its water through perspiration. Daily water turnover for sedentary individuals living in a temperate environment is typically about 2–3L per day, but may be more or less than this for some individuals. Since it is not uncommon to lose 1–5L of water when exercising it is not

WIND SPEED MPH	WHAT IT EQUALS ON EXPOSED FLESH											
	50	40	30	20	10	0	–10	–20	–30	–40	–50	–60
	WHAT THE THERMOMETER READS (DEGREES F)											
40	26	10	–6	–21	–37	–53	–69	–85	–100	–116	–132	–148
35	27	11	–4	–20	–35	–49	–67	–82	–98	–113	–129	–145
30	28	13	–2	–18	–33	–48	–63	–79	–94	–109	–125	–140
25	30	16	0	–15	–29	–44	–59	–74	–88	–104	–118	–133
20	32	18	4	–10	–25	–39	–53	–67	–82	–96	–110	–121
15	36	22	9	–5	–18	–36	–45	–58	–72	–85	–99	–112
10	40	28	16	4	–9	–21	–33	–46	–58	–70	–83	–95
5	48	37	27	16	6	–5	–15	–26	–36	–47	–57	–68
CALM	50	40	30	20	10	0	–10	–20	–30	–40	–50	–60

Little danger if properly clothed	Danger of freezing exposed flesh	Great danger of freezing exposed flesh

Wind chill factor chart.

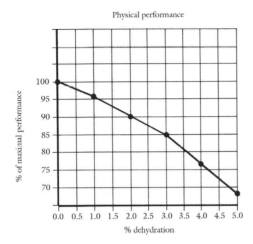

Reduction in performance with dehydration.

difficult to enter the stage of dehydration. Athletes training intensively in hot climates can lose 10–15L of fluid per day, with most of the increase coming from sweat losses. This figure represents about 25–30% of total body water (Maughan and Shirreff, 2004).

The combination of dehydration and high body temperature can cause a number of physiological problems such as:

- a reduction of blood volume
- an increase in the breakdown of liver and muscle glycogen (a sugar used for muscle energy) and
- the inability of the body effectively to pass certain electrolytes across the cell membranes.

While people who exercise should replace 100% of the fluids lost, it is seldom done. The normal person will replace only about 50% during the exercise period. Dehydration of 4% of the body's weight will reduce endurance by 30% in temperate conditions but by as much as 50% when the weather is very warm.

The relationship between dehydration and loss of aerobic capacity is graphically represented in a straight line. Players and coaching staff must be encouraged to try to maintain players' hydration. How can this be monitored? As ever, this starts at the pre-match meal. Players should be encouraged to inspect their urine as they pass it. It should be as clear as water. This diluted urine is a good indication of good hydration. Players should be given adequate fluids on the way to, and in, the dressing room so that the normal fluid loss – in breathing, passing urine – is continually replaced. This should, of course, go on whilst the team is warming up on the pitch.

There are guidelines on dehydration. The American College of Sports Medicine recommends daily weighing of players at pre-season camps, and both before and after play sessions. This gives an indication of fluid loss; 1kg weight loss equals 1L water loss. When results are fed back to the players, they soon learn to realise, without being weighed, how dehydrated they are.

Problems Caused by Heat

Heat cramps

These are generally found in the cramping of the legs, arms or abdomen. The victim will be able to think clearly and will have a normal rectal temperature. The treatment is to give fluids with salt and possibly other minerals, such as are found in most fluid replacement drinks. Heat cramps are particularly common among exercisers who are not yet in good physical condition and who are participating on warm days. There should be no problem in returning to activity the next day.

Heat exhaustion

This is generally caused by a lack of fluid or salts in the body. Water depletion heat exhaustion is caused by insufficient water intake or excessive sweating. The symptoms may include: intense thirst, weakness, chills, fast breathing, impaired judgement, nausea, a lack of muscular coordination or dizziness, or both. If untreated it can develop into heat stroke, with a rectal temperature of over 104°F (40°C). The immediate treatment is to give water or an electrolyte replacement drink – a typical sports drink. When the case is severe it may require intravenous fluid replacement. The skin will generally feel cool and somewhat moist.

Salt depletion heat exhaustion

This appears to be similar to heat cramps. It can occur when large volumes of sweat are replaced only with water. If a great deal of salt was lost in the perspiration it can affect muscle functioning. It is most likely to occur during the first five to ten days of exercising in the heat. The symptoms may include: vomiting, nausea, inability to eat, diarrhoea, a headache (particularly in the front of the head), weakness, a lower body temperature and muscle cramps. Weight loss and thirst are not symptoms of this problem.

Heat stroke

Heat stroke can be caused by heavy exercise just as it can by high air temperature. It is a very serious condition that can affect many of the organs, and occurs when the interior organs of the body are heated above 106°F (42°C). At this temperature protein begins to break down. Enzymes are affected as are the cell walls. When the cells cannot function effectively, organ functioning is impaired.

In addition to a body temperature in excess of 104°F (40°C) there can be a rapid pulse (100 to 120 beats per minute) and low blood pressure. There may also be confusion, weakness, fatigue, delirium, or the victim may lapse into a coma. In contact sports, the confusion that may be exhibited is often mistaken for a head injury. The skin colour is greyish, indicating poor circulation, and it will be clammy. There may or may not be sweating. The pupils of the eyes may be very small.

Treatment requires the immediate cooling of the body. Do not wait for the hospital to treat the victim: it may be too late. Use ice packs to the neck and groin. Full immersion in a tub of cold water is better. Anyone who has experienced heat stroke should not return to activity for at least a week or two.

Reducing the Risk of Heat-Related Problems

Athletic trainers often require that athletes regain 80% of their fluid loss from a session before leaving the locker room. So if an athlete weighed 150lb (68kg) before a practice and 146lb (67kg) afterward, the trainer could require that the athlete take in enough fluids to bring the weight back to slightly over 149lb before leaving the facility. Some sport scientists recommend replenishing the liquids lost with one-and-a-half times the amount lost because additional water will be lost through urine. Fluids or food consumed after training must include sufficient electrolytes – especially sodium – to replace the losses in sweat, although short-term deficits can be tolerated. Food can also make a major contribution to water intake: the water content of a tomato (95%), for example, is higher than that of a cola drink (89%). If large volumes of plain water are consumed, urine production is stimulated because of the fall in the plasma osmolality and sodium concentration.

Dehydration due to excessive heat and/or inadequate fluid intake can cause serious heat-related illnesses. A sudden change in the heat or humidity at practice sessions, or travel to a warmer or more humid climate to compete, can cause problems. A player from the UK who travels to India, Egypt or the Caribbean to compete in a soccer game would probably take ten days to two weeks to acclimatize to the warmer or more humid climate.

Among the changes that will probably occur in a high heat environment are:

- a reduced heart rate (because there is less need for blood to heat the skin, resulting in less blood flow to the skin
- an increase in the amount of blood plasma
- increased sweating, perspiring earlier when exercising
- increased salt losses, and
- the psychological adjustments made to the experience of greater heat and humidity.

in the blood and other tissues. These make the body less efficient and, in some cases, can result in serious sickness or even death. To keep the body hydrated there should be frequent breaks for fluid intake. However, even frequent breaks seldom give an exerciser enough fluid. A person's thirst does not signal the true need for fluids.

The ingredients of sweat change during exercise. At the beginning there are a number of salts excreted. Sodium chloride (common table salt) as well as potassium, calcium, chromium, zinc, and magnesium salts can be lost. The initial sweat contains most of these salts but as the exercise continues, the amount of salts in the sweat may be reduced because some of the body's hormones come into play. Aldosterone, for example, conserves sodium for the body. Consequently the longer we exercise the more our sweat resembles pure water. Just as we vary in nearly every other area, we sweat differently. Some players sweat more or lose more salts than others. The 'salt sweaters' are more likely to develop muscle cramps, so they must be aware that they will need extra salt through the consumption of sport drinks or by adding some extra salt to their meals. However, most of us have plenty of sodium in our daily diets. A normal diet replaces all of the necessary elements lost in sweat for many athletes. Drinking a single glass of orange or tomato juice replaces all or most of the calcium, potassium and magnesium lost.

HYDRATION

Adequate fluid is essential to the functioning of an efficient body. When body fluids are reduced by sweating, less fluid is available

Rehydration

Daily water turnover for sedentary individuals living in a temperate environment is typically about 2–3L per day, but may be more or less than this for some individuals. Athletes training intensively in hot climates can lose 10–15L of fluid per day, with most of the increase coming from sweat losses. This figure represents about 25–30% of total body water. Although such high sweat rates are uncommon, they show that very high fluid losses can be tolerated, provided that a suitable rehydration plan is followed.

Failure to replace sweat losses between training sessions or rounds of a competition will severely impair exercise capacity and will increase the risk of heat-related illness.

Although athletes may learn to tolerate dehydration in the sense that they complain less, their bodies do not seem to adapt to dehydration. Athletes may need to change their normal habits to drink what they need, rather than what they want. Taste is important for many, so a pleasing drink may make some athletes drink more.

Cold Weather Problems

Exercise in cold weather also requires adequate fluid intake. Athletes need to warm the air they breathe and their bodies are still producing heat. They will tend to produce more urine. These factors require them to take in more fluid. Otherwise, the body will feel colder because the blood will not have sufficient volume to warm the skin effectively with the heat that it picks up from the exercising muscles.

Proper Hydration

Fluid replacement drinks vary considerably in their content. Water, the most needed element, is slowed in its absorption if the drink contains other elements such as salts and some forms of sugar. Water alone is therefore sometimes the recommended drink for fluid replacement – and it is certainly the least expensive. For those who want to replace water and sugars for energy the best drinks are those which contain glucose polymers (maltodextrins). So when using fluid replacement drinks, check the label then buy what is needed: salts and/or sugars. Both caffeine (coffee, tea, and cola drinks) and alcohol dehydrate the body so should be avoided.

There is no question that adding carbohydrates, such as glucose, fructose or maltodextrins, is highly effective in replacing the body's fuel. In a study of marathon runners given either a high carbohydrate drink or a placebo every fifteen minutes during a run, those

Blueness or puffiness of the skin	Apathy
Drowsiness	Uncontrolled shivering
Vague, slow, slurred, thick speech	Poor judgement, dizziness, blackouts, unconciousness
Apparent exhaustion	Frequent stumbling, lurching gait
Decreased heart and respiratory rate, weak and irregular pulse	Memory lapses, disorientation, mental confusion

Signs of hypothermia.

	Heat Cramps
SIGNS AND SYMPTOMS	1. Severe muscle cramps in arms or legs.
	2. Muscle cramping may occur in the abdominal muscles.
	3. Profuse sweating.
MANAGEMENT OF HEAT CRAMPS	1. Immediate cessation of exercise.
	2. Consumption of fluids, either water or some type of solution containing sodium chloride (table salt) at a concentration of about one teaspoon of salt per 2 pints (1 litre) of water.
	3. Static stretching of the involved muscles.

	Heat Exhaustion
SIGNS AND SYMPTOMS	1. Moist, clammy skin.
	2. Muscle fatigue (general).
	3. Nausea or related gastrointestinal distress.
	4. Dizziness and occasionally loss of consciousness.
	5. Increased respiratory rate and rapid pulse.
	6. Body temperature ranging from 101°F to 104°F (38.5°C to 40°C).
MANAGEMENT OF HEAT EXHAUSTION	1. Immediate cessation of exercise.
	2. Move the athlete to a cool place.
	3. Place the athlete in a supine position, with legs elevated 8–12in (20–30cm).
	4. Loosen clothing and cool the athlete with wet towels or ice packs.
	5. If the athlete is not fully recovered within 30 minutes, seek medical attention.

	Heat Stroke
SIGNS AND SYMPTOMS	1. Sweating may or may not.
	2. Hot, dry skin.
	3. Mental confusion and possible loss of conciousness.
	4. Gastrointestinal distress, including nausea, vomiting and cramping.
	5. Severe motor disturbances and loss of co-ordination.
	6. Rapid and strong pulse.
MANAGEMENT OF HEAT STROKE	1. This is a medical emergency: summon EMS.
	2. Move the athlete to a cool dry place.
	3. Wrap the athlete in wet sheets or towels, or place cold packs in areas with abundant blood supply, e.g., neck, armpits, head and groin.
	4. Treat for shock and monitor temperature. Do not allow body temperature to drop below 102°F (39°C).
	5. Keep the athlete in a semi-seated position.

Prevention of Heat Disorders
1. Consume fluids and avoid dehydration when participating in activities in warm and humid environments. Experts recommend the consumption of 0.5 pint (0.25 litres) of water every 30 minutes of activity.
2. Avoid heavy exertion during times of extreme environmental conditions, especially when the temperature is above 95°F (35°C) and there is high humidity.
3. Wear proper clothing. Remember that restrictive garments can impair circulation of air, thus reducing the evaporation of sweat. Be aware that dark colours on uniforms and helmets may facilitate heat build-up.
4. Be reminded that fitness has a positive effect on the ability to function in extreme conditions. The process of developing a tolerance to extremes of climate, or acclimatization, normally requires a period of weeks.

Prevention and management of heat-related disorders.

receiving the high carbohydrate drink were able to keep the blood sugar glycogen much higher during and after the run (Nieman *et al.*, 1997).

While water is often recommended as the drink to replace lost perspiration, there are times when some electrolytes (sodium, potassium, etc.) must be replaced. Soccer players working in the heat of the summer sun in warm climates will probably need extra electrolytes. In a study testing whether sodium or sugars (glucose) were more important, it was found that the sugars were more important in fluid replacement beverages. Sodium is often a necessary ingredient for rehydration, but sugars are essential for faster hydration. The sodium content should be about 50–80 mmol per litre of sodium. The sugar content is recommended to be about 4% glucose and 4% fructose (Gisolfi *et al.*, 1993).

When soccer players are exercising for more than fifteen minutes or exercising in the heat they must be conscious of the need for fluid. In such situations it may be wise to eat a diet higher than normal in potassium and, depending on the amount of sweat, some extra sodium. Drinks with extra electrolytes, such as V-8 juice or orange juice, or a sport drink with these elements, might be consumed. Even a minimal level of dehydration (less than 2% loss of body weight due to perspiration) impairs the cardiovascular and the heat-regulating abilities of the body. Even when exercising for less than an hour, fluid replacement is essential.

AIR POLLUTION

Air may be free, but it is a limited resource. Normal air contains 21% oxygen, and when the percentage of oxygen in the air drops to 16%, the brain is affected. Life cannot be supported if the oxygen level drops to 6%. Vegetation takes in the carbon dioxide that we breathe out, then gives off the oxygen that we breathe in. This is one part of the process called photosynthesis, and is one reason why forest preservation is so vital. An acre of beech trees in a forest consumes 2,000lb (907kg) of carbon dioxide while giving out 1,500lb (650kg) of oxygen each day.

Air pollution is nothing new. In the thirteenth century, it was against the law to burn coal in London while Parliament was in session. Air pollution comes from natural sources such as volcanoes and swamps, and also from dumps and mining. Carbon monoxide, a toxic gas, comes from the smoke of any kind of fire. Chlorine gas and hydrocarbons are also air pollutants.

As humans produce more and more pollutants, which escape into the atmosphere, natural processes become unable to clean all of the air, and concern about pollutants becomes urgent. According to the National Air Pollution Control Administration, 42% of air pollution comes from transportation (cars and lorries); 21% from fuel combustion in homes; industrial processes contribute 14%; forest fires contribute 8%; solid waste disposal 5%; and other sources 10%.

Motor vehicles burn more than 600 million gallons of petrol *each day* in the USA. This burning increases nearly all the pollutants in the air. In a city such as Los Angeles, cars and lorries produce 45 tons of particulates, 585 tons of nitrogen oxide, 35 tons of sulphur dioxide, and 9,775 tons of carbon monoxide daily. Aircraft add an additional 19 tons of nitrogen oxide and 190 tons of carbon monoxide to that city's air.

Sulphur compounds are a particular problem. Sulphur dioxide plus oxygen in the air becomes sulphur trioxide, which is more irritating than sulphur dioxide (SO_2). The sulphur trioxide then combines with water vapour in the air to become sulphuric acid. Coal, which is up to 5% sulphur, is a major contribution to the sulphur dioxide content of the air. The sulphuric acid is bad enough on our lungs and on painted surfaces but it is then picked up through convection and becomes an ingredient in the acid rain that has become quite common in northern latitudes.

Carbon monoxide (CO) is released by burning, especially burning petrol and smoking cigarettes, and is picked up by haemoglobin in the blood. Haemoglobin is an iron compound in the red blood cells that transports oxygen from the lungs to the muscles and other tissues. However, if carbon monoxide is available in the air, haemoglobin prefers it to oxygen. The haemoglobin is then rendered useless in transporting necessary oxygen to the tissues. The heart must work harder and the blood pressure is increased. This strains the heart by making it work unnecessarily.

Carbon monoxide in the blood is increased while driving a car, standing on a busy road, smoking, or just living in the city. In central Los Angeles, carbon monoxide has been measured as high as 400 parts per million. At 600 parts per million, drowsiness occurs, and at 1,000 parts per million can induce coma. Exposure to carbon monoxide of 1% in the air for five minutes can be fatal.

Among the symptoms of carbon monoxide poisoning (high carbo-oxi-haemoglobin levels) are headache, nausea, dizziness and a lack of muscular coordination. Such poisonings are most likely to occur to people who work near cars, such as mechanics, police officers and car park attendants, or people who smoke.

In a study done at the University of California in the 1960s, rats exposed to carbon monoxide levels comparable to city motorways developed a preference for alcohol over pure water, sugar water, or saccharin water. The control group of rats breathing normal air preferred pure water. Is it possible that smog contributes to alcoholism?

Nitrogen oxides are a family of highly reactive gases that include nitrogen dioxide (NO_2) and nitric oxide, which form when fuel is burned at high temperatures. They emanate principally from motor vehicle exhaust and stationary sources such as electric utilities and industrial boilers. Oxides of nitrogen play a role in the atmospheric reactions that produce ground-level ozone pollution. In the lungs, oxides of nitrogen can also generate free radicals, particularly NO_2, which appears to be negligible during normal activities, but at high exercise intensities the impact remains unclear.

Ozone (O_3) is a type of molecule of oxygen that performs the necessary function of filtering out some of the harmful radiation of the sun. This occurs in the upper atmosphere eight to thirty miles (13–48km) above the earth's surface. In the last thirty years there has been a huge loss of ozone in the stratosphere due to air pollutants such as aerosols. Exposure to elevated ozone concentrations has been reported to give rise to symptoms that include cough, chest pain, difficulty in breathing, headache, eye irritation and a decrease in forced expiratory volume in one second. All of these effects are likely to impact upon performance.

Chlorofluorocarbons (CFCs) from aerosols and the freon used in air conditioning gases deplete the earth's protective ozone layer. Every drop in ozone increases the amount of ultraviolet (UV) light that reaches the ground, increasing skin damage and the risk of skin cancer. It also increases the incidence of cataracts.

But in the lower atmosphere, ozone is an irritating element of smog. It breaks down some membranes in plants, causing them to lose water and nutrients, and eventually die. This happens when the concentration of ozone is 1–5 parts per 10 million parts of air. Rats exposed to ozone develop lesions in their bronchial tubes and lungs but do not seem to develop cancer (Boorman *et al.*, 1994).

Various studies have indicated that some people may be able to build a tolerance to the negative effects of ozone. In general, residents of Los Angeles have developed some capacities for rebuilding lung tissues damaged by the pollutant. On the other hand, people with chronic emphysema, respiratory diseases, or people who have not been exposed to smog (such as many residents of Canada) do not have such abilities.

The possible effects of air pollution are many. Lung cancer and emphysema are the most common that come to mind; but increased carbon monoxide levels certainly make the blood less effective in transporting oxygen to the muscles. The effect of breathing air pollutants is increased when soccer players must breathe more deeply to get the oxygen to their lungs as they exercise. This deeper breathing brings in more of the pollutants, increases the carbon monoxide in the blood and increases the risk for lung diseases later in life.

Recommendations

Athletes must be adequately hydrated. They must understand the importance of this for both their health and their soccer performance. Some sports drinks will help the athlete to replace carbohydrate and electrolytes.

Exercising in air-polluted environments should be avoided or reduced. Usually exercising in the morning and on the weekends will have a lesser negative impact because air pollution tends to increase during the day on work days and there is less motor traffic at the weekends.

Additionally, because free oxygen radicals are released by both air pollution and normal exercise, antioxidants should be taken. Beta carotene and vitamins C and E are the most commonly available.

CHAPTER 11
Ergogenics and Drugs

Ergogenic means 'work enhancing' or 'energy producing'. So ergogenic aids are whatever facilitates progress toward strength or bulk development or aerobic or anaerobic work. They can range from legal vitamin pills to illegal steroids.

Supplementation with legal substances can help to improve performance, to avoid fatigue, or to live longer. This supplementation is generally for a specific purpose. One supplement may work on the 'fast twitch' (type II) muscle fibres, which are used in weightlifting and sprinting (*see* Chapter 3). Another may work on the slow twitch (type I) fibres, which are used in endurance activities. Still another can provide the necessary building blocks for bones and other tissues. Another can make the blood more effective. Supplements can affect an athlete's chance of injury by increasing the risk, as steroids do, or decreasing the risk, for example by using an effective sports drink during and after exercise.

It is generally accepted that some vitamin and mineral supplements may help you live longer and better, especially those which include antioxidants. On the other hand, some supplements may cost a great deal but do little or nothing. A recent study of a certain dietary supplement advertised as beneficial for sports people found no beneficial effects on performance or recovery in trained athletes. The scientific findings were quite different from the advertising claims.

AIDS TO BUILDING MUSCLE

Building muscle requires working effectively with resistance exercises. It is also vital to have a diet with sufficient amounts of high-quality protein. Protein pills are expensive, and better (and cheaper) protein is to be had from egg whites, skimmed or powdered milk, fish and skinless chicken. Certain vitamins and minerals are also essential in building muscle tissue.

Amino Acids

Amino acids, the building blocks of protein, are often used as supplements to make certain that there is sufficient protein in the body to develop the desired muscle bulk. The advantage of the amino acids over a high-protein meal is that the meal generally includes a great deal of fat, while the amino acids are fat-free. A cheaper and better source of high protein would be dry non-fat milk powder or low-fat cottage cheese. It is important to know what an athlete's protein intake is before he or she embarks on a high-protein plan.

The branched-chain amino acids (BCAA) valine, leucine, isoleucine make up 30–40% of muscle protein. It has been thought that supplementing with them might help to build muscle protein and to increase endurance, or both. While most amino acids are metabolized by the liver, the low levels of the necessary enzyme for breaking down BCAA in the liver force them into the skeletal muscles where more of the necessary enzyme is found. Exercise increases the amount of this enzyme in the muscle so more of the BCAA can be utilized. However, this does not increase one's endurance. There is also a question as to whether it can increase muscle size through the build-up of muscle protein. There is no strong evidence to support the hypothesis that BCAAs as supplements will help athletic performance. Still there seems to be a great deal of interest in the amino acids that are branch chained.

Of the branched chain amino acids, leucine has been the most thoroughly investigated because its oxidation rate is higher than that of isoleucine or valine. Leucine also stimulates protein synthesis in muscle and is closely associated with the release of the factors that allow for the synthesis of glucose from molecules which are not carbohydrates (called gluconeogenic precursors), such as amino acids, lactates and the glycerol part of fat molecules. Leucine makes up about 5–10% of body proteins.

The blood levels of leucine drop after exercise, from 11 to 33% after aerobic exercise, from 5 to 8% after anaerobic exercise and by about 30% after strength exercises. In a Finnish study using power-trained athletes on a diet including the generally recommended protein intake of 1.26g of protein per kilogram of body weight, in a speed and strength programme after five weeks there was a 20% reduction of leucine. Leucine supplementation of 50mg per kilogram of body weight per day, as a supplement to the daily protein intake of 1.26g per kilogram of body weight

per day, appeared to prevent the decrease in the serum leucine levels in power-trained athletes (Pitkanen, 2003). The investigators suggest that the current recommended dietary intake of leucine be increased from 14mg per kilogram of body weight per day to a minimum of 45mg for sedentary individuals, and more for those participating in intensive training in order to optimize rates of whole body protein synthesis.

While consumption of BCAAs, which are 30–35% leucine, before or during endurance exercise has been suggested as a way to prevent, or decrease, the rate of protein breakdown, the studies have not shown whether it will affect an athlete's performance. It might have a sparing effect on muscle sugar breakdown and the reduction of muscle glycogen stores, but the studies are not unanimous. In one study leucine supplementation (200mg per kilogram of body weight) taken fifty minutes before anaerobic running exercise had no effect on performance. However, in another study, during five weeks of strength and speed training, dietary supplementation of the leucine metabolite beta-hydroxy-beta-methylbutyrate (HMB) at 3g a day, to athletes undertaking intensive resistance training exercise, resulted in an increased deposit of muscle and an accompanying increase in strength. Muscle proteolysis (muscle protein breakdown) was also decreased with HMB. Additionally there were lower blood levels of enzymes, which would indicate muscle damage, and an average 50% decrease in plasma essential amino acid levels.

Most studies of leucine supplementation have included the other BCAAs. There have been relatively few studies looking only at leucine. One study, which included 76% leucine as part of a BCAA study, indicated a reduction of fats in and around the organs and a higher level of performance by the athletes.

Another amino acid, tryptophan, is associated with both fatigue and sleep. Either leucine alone or the three BCAAs can reduce the amount of tryptophan in the blood and possibly reduce fatigue. Still another amino acid, glutamine, has been considered to have the potential to slow muscle protein loss.

In spite of these isolated bits of research, one of the leading investigators in the world states that 'in contrast to the claims made on sport nutrition products, branched-chain amino acids do not improve endurance performance; the evidence that glutamine supplements may improve immune function is rather weak, and the available commercial supplements contain too little arginine to increase growth hormone levels. No studies have been performed to investigate the claim that tyrosine supplements can improve explosive exercise' (Wagenmakers, 1999). These criticisms are amplified by Williams (1999), who has written that 'Although current research suggests that individuals involved in either high-intensity resistance or endurance exercise may have an increased need for dietary protein, the available research is either equivocal or negative relative to the ergogenic effects of supplementation with individual amino acids.'

So the jury is definitely out on the need for supplementation with specific amino acids. The more common advice is that if additional protein is needed in the diet, egg whites, non-fat milk and fish are the best sources of complete proteins. Normally, athletes on high-calorie well-balanced diets get enough total protein. Those on low-calorie diets or those who are vegans (vegetarians who do not eat milk products or eggs) might profit from informed supplementation.

High-carbohydrate Foods

High-carbohydrate foods should be taken before or immediately after a workout to replace the glycogen stores in the muscles. Those products with simpler glucose molecules (short-chain glucose polymers, maltodextrins) seem more effective in replacing muscle glycogen than the products that use table sugar (sucrose) as the carbohydrate source.

Vitamin and Mineral Supplements

Vitamin and mineral supplements are often used by athletes to make certain that they are getting enough of the necessary vitamins and minerals. The one-a-day time-release type is best. Supplementing with the antioxidants is also recommended. Since free oxygen radicals are produced continually by the body, and their production is increased by exercise and air pollution, it is wise to take additional vitamins C and E, selenium and beta carotene. Other antioxidants are found in grape skins and other fruits.

Increasing Muscle Size Through Strength Training

Testosterone, the male hormone, is primarily responsible for muscle growth. It has been shown that strength work, in itself, increases testosterone. For example, heavy strength training responses (4 sets of 10-repetition maximum squats with 90 seconds rest between sets) increases the amount of total testosterone, free testosterone and the insulin-like growth factor.

Illegal Substances

Steroids

There are several kinds of steroid hormones in the body. They are composed of fats and each has a particular chemical make-up. The anabolic steroids are associated with muscle development. Anabolic or androgenic steroids are analogues of the male hormone testosterone. Both types have a core 17-carbon steroid chemical structure that gives them anabolic (protein building) and androgenic (masculinizing) properties. Studies were developed to separate the anabolic from the adrogenic effects but this has been only partially accomplished. The androgenic effects of the hormones produced in the body are the development of the male reproductive system and secondary sexual characteristics.

The various steroids may stimulate muscle growth for those who are working with heavy resistance exercises, but they have quite negative effects, which may vary from drug to drug. This is why they are not allowed in sports. Among the potential problems are:

- brittle bones that frequently break
- high blood pressure
- breast tenderness
- liver damage
- sperm count reduction
- a reduction of the size of the testicles
- occasionally death.

For athletes one of the major problems has been damage to the connective tissues. Studies show tendon damage in animals that are fed steroids and made to exercise. Steroid users, who usually deny the possibility of heart damage through steroid use, will gener-ally accept the fact of tendon damage. Steroids cause the body to make abnormal collagen, so they weaken tendons more than other body parts. The muscle–tendon junction is especially weakened.

The pathological effects on collagen are a major reason why steroid users age so quickly; their unnaturally wrinkled faces are due to the abnormal collagen deposited in their skin.

Teenage boys, who take steroids to develop bodies that they think are more attractive to girls, may speed up their secondary sex characteristic development, but their bones harden too early. This can stunt their growth.

The negative effects of the anabolic steroids far outweigh any benefits. That is why they are illegal.

When steroids are taken, the hypothalamus, the part of the brain that monitors and controls all hormone production, picks up the signal that there are too many male hormones in the body. It may then signal the pituitary gland, the adrenals, and the testicles to stop producing their hormones. When the steroid user stops using, the body may have difficulty adjusting to making its own hormones again. Many people who have been on steroids have also noted an increase in their aggressiveness. This is probably due to the androgens such as testosterone and similar substances.

Steroids must be prescribed by a physician. However, since they are available on the black market, most are obtained illegally. To compound the problem, many bodybuilders have taken ten to twenty times the amount that would have given them maximum results. They have mistakenly assumed that if one is good, more is better, when in fact an excess sometimes slows the growth and strength-development process.

While there is no question that anabolic steroids add muscle bulk, there is a question as to just how much more one can gain with steroids rather than good food. The few studies in this area indicate very little difference. So anyone interested in strength and bulk gain should forget about steroids and just work hard, get the proper nutrition, and take sufficient rest.

Harmful effects of steroid hormones

- Leukaemia (blood cancer), liver cancer, and other liver problems
- Premature closing of the growth plates in the bones, stopping growth in height
- Bone brittleness, often resulting in breaks
- Decreasing testicle size in men (and reduced reproductive capacity)
- Breast soreness and enlargement (males)
- High blood pressure
- Lower amounts of high density lipoprotein (HDL) in the blood, which increases the possibility of hardening the arteries
- Increased blood clotting
- Abnormal enlargement of the heart
- Risk of sudden cardiac arrest
- Kidney damage
- Liver inflammation, which can result in cancer
- Impaired thyroid and pituitary functions
- Increase in nervous tension
- Problems with the prostate gland
- Impotence (males)
- Oily skin
- Skin rashes and acne
- Increased body hair
- Thinning hair on scalp
- Gastrointestinal problems
- Muscle cramps or muscle spasms
- Headaches
- Dizziness or drowsiness
- Nosebleeds

Human growth hormone

Considered to be the best steroid, HGH has been shown to increase the size of genetically underdeveloped muscles in animals and humans. In some studies of people with genetically caused underdeveloped musculature, an increase in muscle size brings with it increased strength. In others, the size increase does not result in increased strength. Because of the potential for increased size and strength, athletes have often used this substance. An Austrian study on the growth hormone (Frische, 1999) indicates that for normal people who are working on resistance training their strength was not improved by the administration of the growth hormone. It seemed that the increased size of the muscle belly was caused by fluid retention or an increase in the connective tissue, not an increase in the protein used in the contracting muscle fibres. These findings were similar in power athletes and weightlifters who did not increase their strength in concentric contraction of the biceps or quadriceps. The body produces its own human growth hormone. The amount it produces is increased during rest periods after strength training workouts.

Increasing Anaerobic Capacity

Anaerobic capacity is the work done before becoming tired and before oxygen begins to be used in the muscular system. Increasing anaerobic capacity can often be done legally. Short bursts of energy that are used in soccer, weightlifting and sprinting are examples of the use of anaerobic energy (that is, without the oxygen which is breathed in). The legal method of increasing an athlete's ability to develop short-term bursts of energy is by the administration of creatine.

Creatine

Creatine is a naturally occurring compound, first discovered in 1835. It is synthesized from the amino acids glycine, arginine and methionine, primarily in the liver, but also in the kidneys and the pancreas. It is essential for muscle functioning. While creatine is naturally occurring and is found in good amounts in both meat and fish, most of it is destroyed in the cooking process. A normal diet provides about one to two grams a day. And the body tends to lose two grams a day (Bemben and Lamont, 2005). Vegetarians have far less. For this reason many researchers recommend that serious athletes in power events, or events which require a surge in power, supplement with this natural body substance.

Creatine plays a vital role as creatine phosphate (phosphocreatine) in regenerating adenosine triphosphate (ATP) in skeletal muscle to energize muscle contraction. The energy source for muscle contractions comes when one phosphate from the ATP breaks off. There is enough ATP in the muscle to last for about one second. With the phosphate (P) in the creatine phosphate supplying the energy to replace the phosphate on the ATP, this anaerobic process can be extended for another six to eight seconds. After that other processes help to resynthesize the ATP. Eventually the aerobic ability of replacing the phosphate on the ATP by the use of oxygen comes into play.

Most people are low in the muscle level of creatine unless they eat huge amounts of raw steak or fish. Taking creatine can increase the amount in the muscle up to the maximum saturation. But the muscle can only hold so much. Taking more than the amount that can be absorbed could potentially be a problem, and although there is no evidence for it yet, some speculate that the kidneys might be affected by high levels of supplementation.

Creatine (Cr) is typically ingested as a monohydrate salt and is widely available for public purchase in supermarkets, nutrition stores, health food stores, and via the Internet and mail-order. Athletes currently use Cr as a potential 'safe and legal' alternative to increase performance, as compared to anabolic steroids. Research has clearly demonstrated that supplementation of 20g/day for several days can increase intramuscular Cr stores by 20–30% in most individuals; 20–40% of this increase will be in the form of phosphocreatine (PCr or CP).

Anaerobic and aerobic sources of energy in middle distance running events

In tests for a 400m run (about 50–55 seconds), an 800m run (about 1½ to 2 minutes) and a 1500m run (about 4–4½ minutes) it was found that for the 400m run about 60% of the energy source was anaerobic, for the 800m it was about 35% and for the 1500m it was 20% or less. Soccer is, on average, 70% anaerobic.

Creatine is found in two forms. Approximately 40% is in the free creatine form (Crfree), while the remaining 60% is in the phosphorylated form, creatine phosphate (CP). The daily turnover rate of approximately 2g per day is met by both food and supplementation and by the body's synthesis of the substance. While more Cr is found in the fast twitch muscles, the slow twitch fibres are able to resynthesize it because of their greater access to oxygen. The only side effect associated with creatine supplementation appears to be a small increase in body mass, which is most likely due to water retention but may be related to increased protein synthesis.

Supplementation is not recommended for the average person, but for the élite-level athlete who uses short bursts of energy, it seems to show promise. Those who supplement Cr must do so correctly. There are two methods.

1   If there is a need to build up the muscle creatine quickly, 5g of creatine monohydrate should be taken four times a day for five days. Taking more will not help, as the excess will merely be excreted in the urine. The tissues can only hold a certain amount. After this initial high dose, 2–5g a day should be taken. After two months the process should be repeated: 20g a day for five days then maintaining the level with 2–5g a day. If the muscle storage of creatine had been reduced over the two-month period it will be brought up to the ideal level by the 20g for five days routine.

2   The second method is to take 3–5g every day. The only side effects reported have been muscle cramping, probably from the increased fluid in the muscle, and some diarrhoea and flatulence. If any danger exists it would probably be from taking more than the recommended dose. There is no evidence that taking more than the recommended amount would help.

Since soccer requires both anaerobic (sprinting) and aerobic (long distance) conditioning, both wind sprints and distance work should be done. While anaerobic conditioning may be aided by creatine supplementation it may help. But the only aids for aerobic conditioning are illegal blood doping, such as the use of the hormone erythropoietin (EPO).

COMMON PSYCHOACTIVE DRUGS

The basic facts about alcohol and tobacco are well known, and players need to be counselled in them. But there are some facts that are not so commonly known.

Psychoactive drugs work by interfering with the neurotransmitters (the chemicals that transmit the nerve impulse from one nerve to another, primarily in the brain). Some neurotransmitters work in the stimulating nerves, others in the relaxing nerves. The different types of psychoactive drugs work differently, some increasing the amount of neurotransmitter, some decreasing it and some mimicking it. With over 200 neurotransmitters in action, it is easy to see how the various drugs exert their effects, causing excitement, calm, hallucinations or sleep. By changing the natural level of normal brain chemicals, psychoactive drugs can negatively affect the nervous system's functions, such as remembering, sleeping, and concentration. They can increase mental illness, anxiety and nervousness.

Creatine supplementation

The American College of Sports Medicine Roundtable made these findings:

- creatine can increase muscle phosphocreatine (PCr) content, but not in all individuals
- a high dose of 20g, which is common in research studies, is not necessary because a longer term use of 3g a day will eventually give the same increase
- ingesting fairly large amounts of carbohydrates at the same time as ingesting the creatine will increase the uptake by the muscles
- exercise performance involving short periods of extremely powerful activity (sprinting, jumping, etc.) can be enhanced, especially during repeated bouts of activity
- Cr supplementation does not increase maximal isometric strength, the rate of maximal force production, nor aerobic exercise performance
- most of the evidence has been obtained from healthy young adult male subjects with mixed athletic ability and training status
- Cr supplementation leads to weight gain within the first few days, likely due to water retention related to Cr uptake in the muscle
- Cr supplementation is associated with an enhancement of strength in strength-training programmes, a response not independent from the initial weight gain, but may be related to a greater volume and intensity of training that can be achieved
- there is no definitive evidence that Cr supplementation causes gastrointestinal, renal, and/or muscle cramping complications
- the potential acute effects of high-dose Cr supplementation on body fluid balance has not been fully investigated
- ingestion of Cr before or during exercise is not recommended.

(Terjung, 2000)

Tobacco

The legal drug tobacco is the second most addictive drug after cocaine. It contains nicotine, which has a well-known effect of raising the blood pressure, which is negative for athletes. It also contains tars, which reduce the ability of the alveoli in the lungs to absorb oxygen from the air. It is the only drug that has both a stimulating 'upper' and a depressive 'downer' effect. Nicotine releases adrenaline, which gives smokers the upper effect and the nicotine acts like a calming brain neurotransmitter in the synapses of the nerves, giving the downer or calming effect. Withdrawal gives the upper effect of a downer withdrawal (such as alcohol or heroin, but not as strong) and the downer effect of withdrawing from an upper drug (such as cocaine). The combination makes withdrawal very difficult.

Alcohol

Alcoholic drink is highly addictive for some people. It also adds unwanted empty calories and can deaden the nerve fibres, which makes it more difficult to coordinate movement effectively. It is also a diuretic so rids the body of water that might be essential for adequate hydration.

Marijuana

The tar in marijuana has the same effect as that in tobacco, with one smoked joint having the same amount of tar as a pack of smoked cigarettes. Since the THC (the major psycho-active ingredient) in marijuana has a half-life of seven to ten days, compared to a half-life of several hours for alcohol, the effects of a smoked joint last for days. Also, the THC is fat-soluble (like LSD and PCP) so it stays in the tissues for weeks; repeated use of the drug increases the amount held in the body. Most drugs are water-soluble so they leave the body more quickly.

Stimulants

Users of drugs such as cocaine, methamphet-amine (speed) and its relative Ecstacy[5] show poor memory and higher than normal body temperature, which is particularly dangerous in warmer climates and can lead to death. They also may increase nausea, depression, blurred vision, muscle tension, nerve damage and a number of other effects which are negative for athletes.

---

5   MDMA or 3,4-methylenedioxymethamphetamine.

CHAPTER 12

Conditioning for Strength and Power

Off season there are several components of the physical skills necessary for soccer to consider, including strength, power, speed, speed endurance, quickness and various agilities. While it was first believed that strength training was the major factor in off-season conditioning, we now realize that strength is only a small part of total conditioning. Off-season conditioning to perform better and to avoid injuries must include those activities shown in the table below, at the recommended percentage of available time.

As has been noted, being in better condition is a major method of avoiding, or at least reducing, injuries. Being in good condition also helps the player to recover faster from injuries. Let us look first at getting into condition to become better soccer players.

Time allotted	Goal	Activity
10 to 25%	Strength training	High resistance, less than ten repetitions, one to three sets, core body strength (abdominals and low back) using stability balls etc.
10%	Power training	Speed and strength combination (about 45% of one repetition maximum done quickly)
10 to 15%	Plyometrics	
	Speed work	
10%		Sprint resistance to increase stride length, uphill sprints, parachutes, towing sleds or tyres
3 to 5%		Sprint assistance to increase stride frequency, downhill running, being towed
15 to 25%		Speed endurance, repeat sprints to develop anaerobic capacities
20 to 30%		Sport-specific movements such as cutting, kicking etc.

Time usage for off-session conditioning.

The same principles and exercises that make better players also help them to reduce, and to recover from, injuries.

While strength is essential for the development of power and speed, these abilities will not develop merely because one becomes stronger. Each ability that players need to develop must be specifically trained. For example, speed is increased by increasing either stride frequency or stride length or both. Strength in the rear of the hips (gluteals), the rear of the thighs (hamstrings) and the calf (triceps suriae) are essential for increasing stride length. Stride frequency requires sufficient strength in the front of the hip and thigh (quadriceps). But strength alone will not make a player faster. For that, power is needed, the combination of strength and speed.

So to increase stride frequency a player can:

* run while being towed (such as by a car)
* do downhill sprints (3–5° decline) or
* do appropriate plyometrics.

For stride length the athlete can:

* run uphill sprints
* tow weights like tyres or running sleds
* do appropriate plyometrics.

No matter how fast players become, if they tire too quickly they will be useless on game day, and being fatigued is a major reason for many injuries. So sprint endurance needs to be developed.

The muscle contractions can be:

* concentric: the muscle shortens as the exercise is performed, the joint angle changes because of the force of the muscular contraction

* isometric: the muscle shortens or tightens but the joint angle does not change, or
* eccentric: the muscles are lengthening under force.

Biceps are in a concentric contraction when curling a weight. Triceps are concentrically contracting when lifting a weight above the head. An isometric contraction occurs when standing in a doorway and pushing outward on the door jambs. The eccentric contraction is common in running. When landing on the toes and the heel comes closer to the ground the calf muscles are in an eccentric contraction. Similarly when the thigh comes forward in a stride, the hamstrings are lengthening and contracting as they begin to start the backward motion of the stride; the backward motion is then a concentric contraction. Hamstring muscle pulls tend to occur at the end of the forward motion of the thigh or at the beginning of the backward movement when the contraction changes from eccentric to concentric.

SPORT-SPECIFIC STRENGTH TRAINING

Traditionally it has been the power lifters who have dominated strength training for sports. What they have done has significantly improved the performances of nearly all athletes. However, sports science has studied the 'sport specificity' of strength and power training and it seems that the exercises should be more sport specific to improve effectiveness. To be sport specific the exercises should consider:

* posture: the position of the body during play

113

- speed
- exact sport movement: such as each type of kicking action.

Posture

Posture refers to the position of the body during the movement, and it has been the subject of much investigation. Top researcher Greg Wilson of Australia, second in the world in power lifting, studied subjects who did maximum bench presses, then from the bench press position threw an unweighted bar as high as possible, then did push ups, then threw a medicine ball as far as possible from a seated position. The same muscles were involved in each activity but there was no transference from one strength exercise to the next. A similar study was reported by America's top exercise scientist, Larry Morehouse (Rasch and Morehouse, 1957). It was also reported in studies by Sam Britten in the 1970s.

Posture is important because the position of the brain when stimulating the muscles is important. Since the strength that a person can generate depends on two factors: the amount of the cross-section of the muscle fibres and the number of those fibres that the person can enervate at one time, we can understand how posture is important in the enervating factor.

Speed

Speed is obviously important, but strength is only a part of speed. Working an exercise fast, at about 40–45% of the one repetition maximum (1 RM), seems to be better than gross strength as shown in a one or ten repetition maximum set. Specific movement as is done during soccer play will develop more strength, power and speed for the game.

Most people are familiar with the typical strength training programmes, so we will begin with the more traditional strength programmes. Since not everyone has weights we will also mention how manual resistance can be used. It makes no difference to the muscles whether they are lifting iron or working against someone else's muscles. At the end of the section there are some sport-specific exercises. Assuming that there is no injury, any strength training exercise will help to some degree. But the sport-specific exercises will help more.

The General Strength Programme

Every athlete should work on a general body conditioning programme before starting the individual exercises. A general body programme would include the following exercises.

- Bench press for upper chest and triceps
- Triceps exercise
- Shoulder (military) press for shoulders and triceps
- Biceps curl
- Squats for legs
- Calf raises
- Hip abduction and adduction
- 'Lats' for upper back
- 'Clean' for legs, back, shoulders and biceps
- Sit-ups for abdominals
- Back extensions for lower back

SPECIFIC PROGRAMME FOR SOCCER PERFORMANCE AND INJURY PREVENTION

While an overall body building programme may be good for all athletes, special exercises can be particularly beneficial to soccer players. However, they may vary for the different field players and they vary considerably for goal-keepers.

Abdominal and lower back strength (core strength) are useful in nearly every activity. Soccer players need strength in every muscle group, particularly the legs.

All soccer players will also need:

- all of the neck exercises (to protect the neck and brain from injury)
- abdominal curl-ups (for speed)
- back extensions
- ankle plantar flexion (for speed, jumping, and running power)
- hip abduction (for moving sideways)
- hip adduction (for moving sideways)
- leg extensions, half squats, or lunges (for leg speed and power)
- eccentric hamstring exercises to reduce the likelihood of pulled hamstrings while running.

The Exercises

Under the heading for each muscle group (such as front of deltoids, or abdominals) several exercises are listed. A programme requires only one of these options.

Neck

Neck injuries can be lifelong problems to soccer players, so they must take special precautions to strengthen the neck. Neck exercises are best done with the hands.

- For the front of the neck have the athlete put the hands on the forehead and push hard against them, flexing the neck forward (below left). This is the most important exercise for heading. A stiff neck will allow the whole body, rather than just the head, to absorb the force of the blow.
- For the back of the neck, put the hands behind the head and extend the neck backward.
- For each side of the neck, put a hand on the side of the head and bend the neck in that direction (below). This is also important for heading.

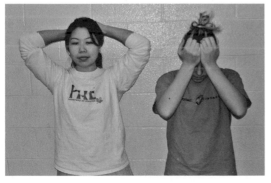

Back and front of neck using manual pressure.

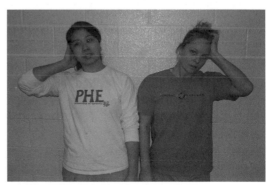

Side of neck using manual pressure.

115

When the neck is moved it is called an isotonic exercise. When the muscles do not move it is called an isometric exercise. Neck exercises should be done both moving (isotonic) and not moving (isometric). When doing the isometric exercise have the player push hard with the head against the hand but the hand should give enough resistance to prevent the head from moving.

Shoulders

The shoulders are involved in every lifting, throwing, and hitting activity as well as in running and walking.

Front of shoulders

The standing forward raise (below) is recommended for goalkeepers, and is also valuable in rehabilitating a shoulder separation.

With a dumbbell in each hand and the palms facing inward, raise the dumbbells forward as high as possible. The exercise can be done with both arms working at the same time or alternately. These muscles help in running so the alternating exercise is better.

Top of shoulders

The standing lateral raise (below) is not a sport-specific exercise for soccer but is useful in shoulder rehabilitation.

Stand with a dumbbell in each hand at the sides of the body, then lift the dumbbells directly overhead with the backs of the hands staying on top of the dumbbells. (Turning the palms up allows the upper chest muscles (pectorals) to join in the work, which is not what is required.)

This exercise also works the upper part of the trapezius, the large muscle in the middle of the upper back, which is used to hold up the shoulders when exercising. Developing this muscle can reduce the chances of muscle tenseness and fatigue during a workout or game.

Back of shoulders

The bent fly or prone fly on a high bench (opposite, top) is not sport specific for soccer.

Lie face down on a bench with dumbbells in each hand, or stand while bending forward

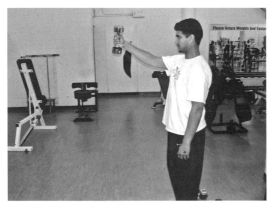

Standing forward raise.

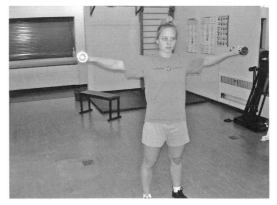

Standing fly (upper deltoids).

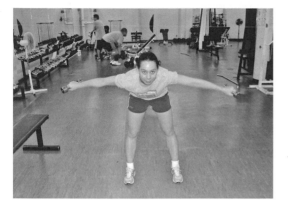

Bent fly (rear deltoids).

at a 90° angle at your waist with your head on a table or against a wall to reduce the pressure on the lower spinal disks. Now raise the dumbbells from directly below the shoulders as far up as they will go. Keep the arms straight.

Abdominals and core strength

Most people are aware of how important it is to have abdominal strength. It helps to keep our bellies tucked in for better posture. In fact the abdominals, along with the lower back, are the two most important areas for strength in our bodies. We call the strength in these areas 'core strength'. In sports the abdominals help to stabilize the hips so they are essential in every action that involves the hip joints: running, jumping and kicking.

In order to attempt to isolate the abdominals, lie on your back and bend the knees as much as possible so that the muscles which flex the hip joint (bringing the thighs forward and upward) will not work as much. Keep the hips (your belt) on the mat when doing an abdominal exercise; whenever the hips are pulled off the mat the hip flexors are working, and this curvature places a higher pressure on the outside of the disks in the lumbar (lower back) region. It causes many problems in later life. The reason that hip flexion exercises can increase the curvature of the spine is that there are some muscles deep inside the pelvis which attach from the lower back bones to the thighbone. As they get stronger they pull in on the lower spine and increase the curvature. You will often see this extreme lower back curve (a lordosis) in female gymnasts.

The abdominal curl-up (below) is done by lying on the floor or on a bench with the knees bent and the arms crossed on the chest or the fingers just touching the head. Curl the shoulders forward until the hips are about to leave the floor. Aim to touch the elbows to the thighs. When the curl-ups are done on an inclined board with the head lower than the feet, the resistance lifted will be increased.

Those working for strength will hold weight plates on the forehead or chest in order to increase resistance. But most players are looking for muscular endurance so that they can hold their tummies in longer. Both are important for football.

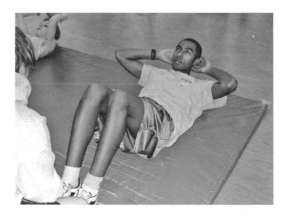

Abdominal curl up.

117

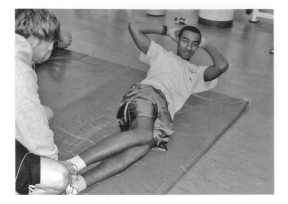

Side sit-up.

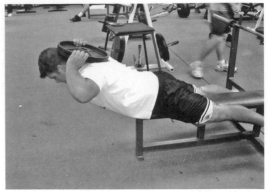

Back extension.

The side sit-up (above) is done to get additional strength for the muscles on the side of the abdominal area (the obliques). The feet have to be held down or hooked under a barbell. Lift the shoulders from the mat or bench. This exercise will work not only the abdominal oblique muscles but also the muscles on one side of the lower back and the rectus abdominis on the side to which one is bending.

Other core exercises can be done balancing on the floor or on a ball. These are usually isometric exercises.

Lower back

Exercises for the lower back are probably the most important for the average person to do because lower back injuries, especially muscle pulls, are so common. The problem is that these muscles do not enhance our general appearance so we often overlook them.

The lower back muscles are particularly important in running because they hold the torso erect. And, of course, they are essential in maintaining good posture because they are the muscles which hold the chest up by rotating the rib cage. They pull the back of the rib cage down, which raises the front of the rib cage and the chest comes up with the ribs.

The back extension (above) can be done on the floor. Just lie face down and raise the shoulders and knees slightly off the floor. Do not make a big arch because hyperextending the spine is not a safe exercise.

An alternative is to use a table or sofa, and lie face down so that the hips are at the edge and the legs are on the table or sofa. The feet are held down. Bend forward up to 90° and then straighten the back, just a bit past the horizontal. If the desired goal is strength, weight plates or a dumbbell can be held behind the head.

Hip flexors

The hip flexors bring the thighs forward so they are essential in any running or jumping activity. Anyone who runs fast must have hip flexor strength, and they are absolutely essential for kicking.

For those who would be susceptible to an excessive lower back curvature, special precautions should be taken. They should keep the connective tissue in their lower backs flexible by doing toe touching exercises while sitting.

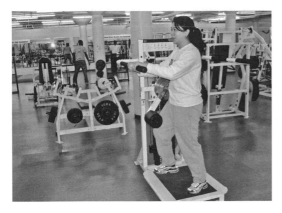

Hip flexion on multi-hip machine.

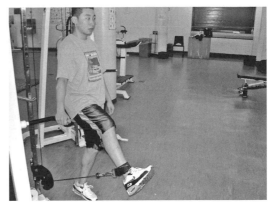

Hip flexion on low pulley.

They should also keep their abdominals strong to reduce the tendency of the front of the hips to drop forward. This would increase the curve of the lower spine.

Hip flexors are exercised when the thigh is brought forward. This can be done:

- hanging or standing
- without weights
- with a weighted boot
- with an ankle attachment to a pulley on a weight machine.

- If a multi-hip machine is available, stand sideways to the machine (above) and with the pad on the front of the thigh lift the pad forward. Get as large a range of motion as possible: from a hyperextended position to a fully flexed position.
- With a weight machine, use the lower pulley and hook the ankles into a handle or use an ankle strap to secure the ankle to the pulley (above right). Raise the leg straight forward.
- While standing, with or without weight boots, brace with the arms then lift one leg forward as high as it will go. Bring it

up slowly.
- Leg lifts are done from the supine position (on the back). Lift one or both legs from the floor to the vertical position. The abdominals will contract isometrically in this, as in all other hip flexion exercises.
- An effective way to gain strength with the manual resistance of a partner is to lie on the side. With the leg straight, extend it backwards as far as possible. The partner will then give manual resistance to the front of the ankle as the leg is brought forward as far as it will go (below).

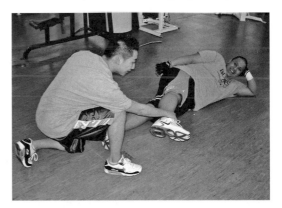

Hip flexion with partner.

Hip extensors

The hip extensor muscles bring the thighs from a forward position back to a straight position such as when you are standing. They will also bring the thighs further back than straight, which is called hyperextension. The hip extensors are the muscles which supply power when a player is running or jumping.

- On a multi-hip machine starting from a hip flexed position, extend the thigh (below).
- Lift the leg forward then have a partner hold the ankle and resist. Lower the leg to the floor.
- While standing, braced for balance, bring one leg backward as far as possible.

- While lying on the side and the leg straight and as far flexed as possible (below), have a partner apply manual resistance to the back of the ankle, and bring the full leg backward as far as possible.

Hip abduction

Hip abduction means moving the leg sideways in a lateral plane. It uses the muscles on the outside of the hips. It is used when a player wants to move laterally while facing ahead. It is important in locomotion because it helps to maintain the torso straight without excessive sideways leaning. It is also used when kicking a ball to the same side, e.g. the right leg kicking right.

- On a multi-hip machine, put the outside of the thigh against the pad and push outward (opposite, top left).
- Lie on the back with a partner holding the outside of the feet or the lower legs. With the partner resisting, push the legs apart as far as they will go (opposite, below).

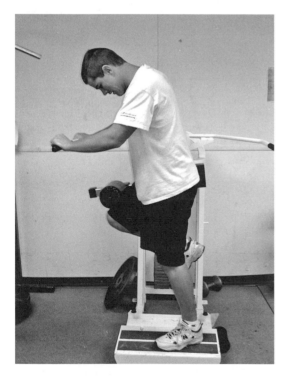

Multi-hip machine hip extension.

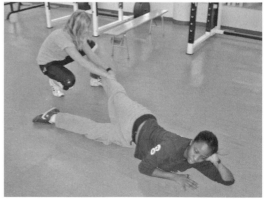

Hip extension with partner.

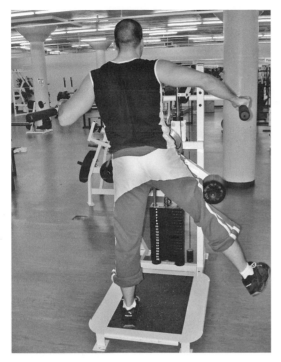

Hip abduction with multi-hip machine.

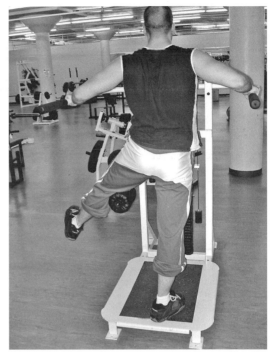

Hip adduction with multi-hip machine.

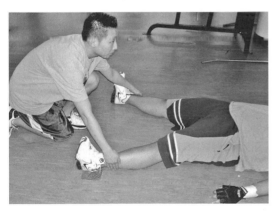

Hip abduction with partner.

- On a machine, use the lower pulley. While standing sideways to the machine at the low pulley station, hook one foot into the handle (or use an ankle strap) and pull the leg away from the machine.

Hip adduction

Hip adduction exercises strengthen the muscles on the inside of the leg (the groin). These muscles are also used in moving laterally and are important for the overall hip strength needed by soccer players. They would also be used in kicking a ball to the opposite side, e.g. the right leg kicking left. Their development may help to prevent groin pulls.

- On a multi-hip machine with the pad on the inside of the thigh squeeze it downward (above).
- With a partner helping, start with legs spread, the partner's hands on the inside of the feet or lower legs to give resistance, and squeeze the legs together (*see* page 122, top left).

121

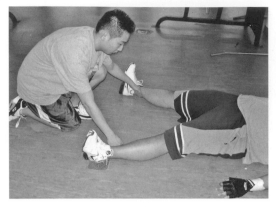

Hip adduction with partner.

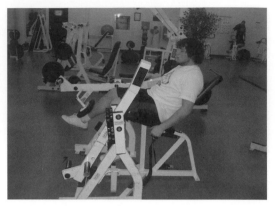

Knee extension on machine.

- On a machine with a low pulley, stand away from the machine sideways to it; with the foot in the handle, squeeze the leg in toward the body pulling the handle away from the machine.

Knee extension

Extending the knee means to straighten it. The leg extensors are used in any running, kicking or jumping action. Some of the major knee extensor muscles also flex the hips, so the following exercises will also strengthen the hip flexors.

- On the leg extension machine, hook the feet under the padded bar and straighten the leg (top right). This exercise can also be done with a weighted boot. Some machines work both legs simultaneously, others work them alternately.
- For manual resistance, sit on a table with a partner having both hands on one ankle (right, below). Try to straighten the leg while the partner gives just enough resistance to allow the movement.

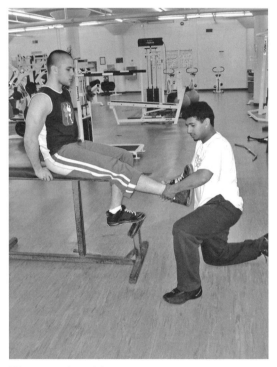

Knee extension with partner.

Knee flexors (leg curls)

The knee flexors bend the knee. They generally work with the hip extensors so are useful in running. If the front of the thighs (the quadriceps or knee extensors) are strengthened, the

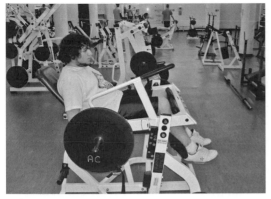

Nordic hamstring exercise on leg flexion machine.

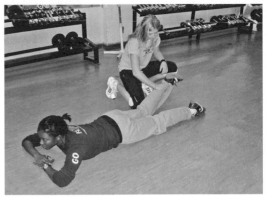

Knee flexion with partner.

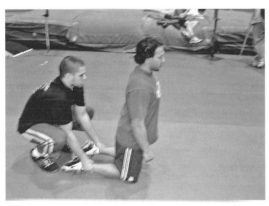

Nordic hamstring exercise with a partner.

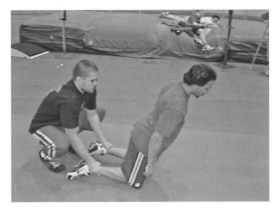

Nordic hamstring exercise, continued.

knee flexors must also be strengthened. This is also the best protection against hamstring pulls, especially when the eccentric aspect of the exercise is emphasized. It is also essential to bring the quadriceps:hamstring strength ratio closer to 1:1, which also reduces the chance of hamstring and knee injuries. The exercise that may be best for reducing hamstring strains is called the Nordic hamstring exercise. It emphasizes the eccentric action, which is the major cause of muscle strains. This is a far better exercise for soccer than the traditional leg curling action (Mjølsnes *et al.*, 2004).

- Kneel on the floor, preferably on a mat. The partner holds the lower legs on the floor. Lower the body forward toward the floor. Resist as long as possible while the torso moves toward the floor. This is the eccentric action. Pull back to an upright position (above, left and right).
- On a leg flexion machine, flex the knee. Return to the extended position slowly to gain more effective eccentric work (top left).
- Lie on the floor, with resistance supplied by a partner's hands on the back of the ankle. Bend the knee. The partner maintains the pressure as the knee is again straightened, for the eccentric work (top right).

123

Ankle plantar flexion

Ankle plantar flexion occurs when the sole of the foot moves closer to the calf muscle. This action occurs when rising up on the toes. This is a key area for strength and power in running and jumping.

- While holding a barbell on the shoulders, rise up on the toes. This is better done with the toes on a riser board because the calf muscle will be gaining flexibility as it stretches down.
- On a weight machine, with the legs straight, allow the weight to bring the ankles back stretching the Achilles tendon, then push the weight out with the calf muscles.
- While holding a table for balance, rise up on one toe (below). This will give the

same resistance as holding a barbell which equals one's body weight and doing the exercise with two legs. For example a 150lb player with a 150lb barbell is lifting 150lb with each calf muscle. With no barbell but only one leg, the calf muscle will still be lifting 150lb.

Using a dumbbell in one hand and doing the exercise with one leg at a time has the same effect as adding double the amount to a barbell and doing the exercise with two legs.

Arm or elbow flexion

Arm flexion occurs when you bend your elbow forward. The biceps curl is the exercise that strengthens this action. The curl can be done with a barbell, a dumbbell, or a set of dumbbells. The biceps are used primarily

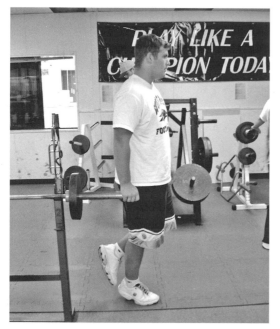

One leg calf rise.

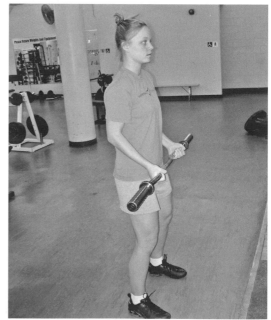

Barbell curl.

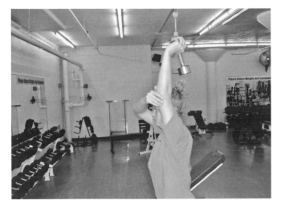

Triceps extension.

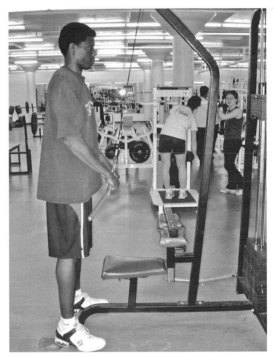

Triceps extension on machine.

by goalkeepers but also aid the field players in running. It is more important for goalkeepers.

- The barbell biceps curl is the most common biceps exercise. With the barbell in the hands (palms up) and the arms extended down, curl the barbell upward (opposite, below). The gripping of the bar will give some isometric strength in the front of the forearms.
- For manual resistance, push down on the palm of one hand while doing a curling action (bringing the hand) up to the shoulder.

Arm (or elbow) extension

These are triceps extension exercises. The triceps are used to straighten the arms. They are therefore used in pushing something away from the body and in throwing. The best exercise for this action is the standing one-arm triceps extension, which gives maximum stretch to the triceps muscle.

- Start with the arm holding the dumbbell extended overhead (above). Steady that elbow with the other hand by holding just below the elbow on the extended arm. (This stops other muscles from coming into play.) Allow the dumbbell to lower as much as possible. This gives maximum flexibility. Then raise the dumbbell overhead for strength.
- On a weight machine use the 'high pulley station'. Grip the bar, and with the elbows at the side, bring the bar down by straightening the arms: a triceps push down (above).
- For simple resistance, bend one arm so that the hand is touching the shoulder, put the hand of the other arm against the wrist of the bent arm. Straighten the bent arm while resisting with the other hand.

Rotator cuff

The four rotator cuff muscles are used when throwing. They rotate the upper arm in the shoulder socket. Goalkeepers should do these exercises.

- Bend forward at the waist. With a dumb-bell in one hand bring it up to hip level while twisting the dumbbell inward.
- While lying on the back with a dumbbell in one hand, the elbow at the side and the forearm at a 90° angle to the body, bring the dumbbell across the chest (below).
- With a low pulley, lie on the floor with the elbow perpendicular to the torso. Pull the arm across the body.
- Standing with the back to a high pulley, with the upper arm extended and parallel to the ground and the lower arm straight up, with the hand grasping the grip on the pulley cable, rotate the arm so that the hand moves through a 180° arc and the lower arm is facing straight down. This is the best exercise. This action can also be done lying on the back with a dumb-bell, or preferably using a low pulley.

The standing exercise is best because the posture is sport specific.

Multiple joint exercises

Bench press

The bench press works the triceps, the front of the shoulders and the upper chest muscles. If any of these muscles are weak, the athlete should isolate the weaker muscles and strengthen them along with working on the bench press. This is not a soccer-specific exercise.

This press is done on a bench rather than on the floor because the arms should be able to come below shoulder level for flexibility. The grip should be wide enough so that when the bar is lowered to the chest, the forearms should be perpendicular to the floor (below).

The back should remain on the bench throughout the exercise. A player who arches will be able to lift a bit more weight because more of the lower pectorals will come into play, but this is considered cheating.

Starting with the bar at arms' length and

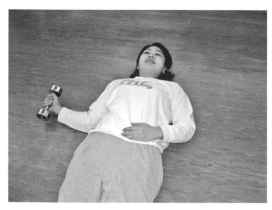

Rotator cuff.

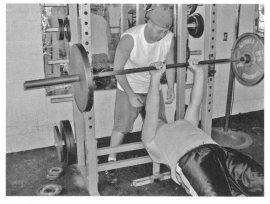

Bench press with spotter.

over the nose, the bar is slowly lowered to the chest then pushed upward. It is important that the bar is not pushed towards the feet or it will be out of control. The proper path of the bar is an arc from a position over the nose, lowered to the area of the nipples, then lifted over the nose. The bar does not go straight up from the chest. Also make certain that the bar is not bounced off the chest.

The exercise can be done with free weights using a rack and a spotter or without a rack and two spotters. The spotters are there to make certain that the athlete does not lose control of the weights and get into danger. Strength training deaths are nearly always caused by bench presses done without a spotter; falling weights can cause fatal choking.

Squats or full leg extensions

Squats or leg extensions work the hip and knee extensors. These are necessary for nearly any running or jumping activity. However, since a squat is a two-legged exercise moving straight up (vertically) it is sport specific for jumping while heading.

- In performing a squat the angle of the knee should not pass the 90° mark. At this point the ligaments, which attach to the cartilages inside the knee, are pulled back in the knee. This makes the cartilages act as fulcrums. The force of the weight downward on this fulcrum increases the stretch on the ligaments in the front of the knee and can stretch them, making the knee structurally weaker and more prone to injury while playing.

If a full squat is done, where the muscles at the back of the thighs and the calf muscles touch,

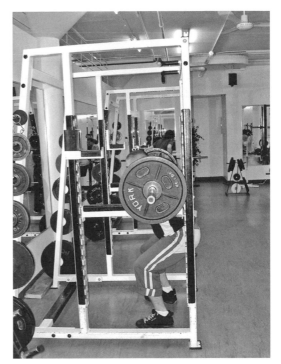

Half squat.

the fulcrum is moved further to the rear and great force is exerted on the ligaments in the front of the knee.

When doing squats in the squat rack be certain that the pins are set so that the hips cannot go too far down and damage the knees.

The most common positions for your feet are either shoulder width with the toes pointed straight ahead or with a wider than shoulder position with the toes pointed slightly outward. The feet should remain flat through the entire lift (above).

It is important to keep the back slightly arched and the head level or up to reduce pressure on the spinal discs. Do not let the torso bend too far forward. Also, do not let the knees get too far ahead of the toes, as then too much weight is being carried forward and balance could be lost. It will also increase the angle of the knee and can result in harmful forces on the ligaments. Bouncing up from the squat position will also increase the strain on the knee ligaments.

During the squatting action the bar should move up and down in a vertical path.

Two variations of the squat are the front squat, with the bar held on the chest, and the hack squat with the bar held behind the back at the level of the buttocks.

- On the leg extension machine there is some built-in safety. The lifter can sit down so that there is not the compressing force of the weight downward on the spinal discs.

On the leg extension machine, as in the squat rack, finish the leg extension with a toe push (ankle plantar flexion). This will make the exercise more like a jump or a sprinting stride.

- A one-legged squat gives the same effect as carrying the body weight on a barbell. Hold on to a table for balance, lift one foot off the floor, and squat with the other leg.

Lunges

This exercise works the same muscles as do the squats, and is popular with world class sprinters.

With a barbell held on the shoulders behind the neck (or dumbbells held at the sides) take a step forward and bend the forward leg into a lunge (above right). The knee should be no farther forward than the toes. Push back up and bring the forward foot back to the starting position. Two smaller steps may be needed to safely return to the starting position.

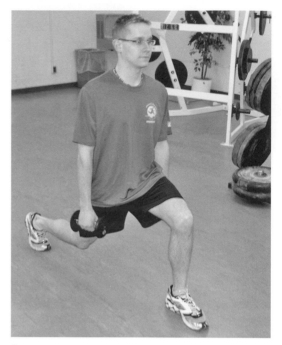

Lunge.

Power clean

The power clean is an essential exercise for competitive weightlifters and is very useful for those, such as soccer players, wishing to develop full body extension power. The exercise works the knee and hip extensors, the ankle plantar flexors, the lower back, the deltoids, the upper trapezius and the biceps. Other muscles are involved to a lesser extent.

The barbell should be on the floor close to the feet. With the feet about shoulder width, bend forward with the back slightly arched and grasp the bar with a wide grip and the palms visible. Start the cleaning action with an explosive 'jump' by straightening the hips, knees, and ankles. At the point where the legs are straightened the bar will be moving fast. Use this velocity to help to pull the bar to chest level. At the top of the movement bring the wrists back and push the elbows forward to allow the bar to settle on the top of the chest. At this point, the knees bend slightly to 'catch' the weight. The bar is then returned to the floor.

Another type of 'clean' ends with the 'high pull' rather than catching the bar on the chest. In the high pull lift the bar as high as possible then return it to the floor without catching it.

The 'hang clean' is often used to teach the power clean. It can also be used for those with weak or injured knees or backs. In the 'hang clean' the barbell is dead lifted to the waist. From this point it is raised to the 'clean' position.

CHOOSING THE WORKOUT SCHEDULE

There are many ways to set up a workout schedule. Exercises can be varied, perhaps by working on squats one day, leg extensions another, and lunges on a third day. The schedule itself might be the same (same weights, same number of repetitions and sets), or can be varied. Here are some ideas for developing a schedule.

- Exercise early in the workout those muscles that need the most work. Research of many years ago indicated that one to three sets of one to three repetitions, or as high as five or six repetitions was best for strength gain. Of course the muscles should be exhausted, or at least very tired, after each set. Recent research has shown that three sets will give about 10% more strength gain than one set. Consequently many professional athletes use only one set, then use the additional time to do other conditioning work, such as speed work or agilities. Well-conditioned weight trainers can generally do more work with each muscle group.

- Rest between sets. Obviously no one can do one set after another without rest. There must be rest between sets, but not for too long. Generally with an isolated movement such as a biceps curl or a triceps exercise one to one-and-a-half minutes is sufficient time for a rest. For a multi-joint exercise such as a press or a squat two to three minutes (maximum) should work.

The fewer repetitions the athlete does to exhaustion, the longer the rest period needed. So a two-repetition maximum set will require a longer rest than a six-repetition maximum set.

- Rest between workouts. Rest is essential for developing muscles because they are damaged in the lifting: especially during the eccentric work. This is the reason that weight training programmes are generally done only every other day while endurance exercises such as swimming or running can be done daily. While most weight trainers must wait 48 hours between workouts, highly trained weight trainers can lift daily if they replace the glycogens (muscle sugars) adequately during the 24-hour rest period. Many lifters rest three days between workouts to recover fully. And after a very hard workout it actually takes up to four days for the muscles to repair and recover.

PART 2

Diagnosis and Treatment

CHAPTER 13

First Aid and Early Treatment

There are a number of preferred methods of treating injuries. Some require special equipment available only at the offices of doctors, physical therapists or athletic trainers. Some emphasize cold treatments, some balance them. In this chapter the method proposed by the British Olympic medical team will be presented (*see* O'Connor *et al.*, 1998). Any injury that seems serious or where the severity is not known should be seen immediately by a competent medical practitioner.

STANDARD TREATMENT FOR INJURIES

The purpose of standard treatment is to stop the swelling and stop the scar tissue from developing. The first area of standard treatment is to apply some type of pressure, such as with an elastic (Ace) bandage.

The application of cold compresses or ice is called for in most injuries in order to stop or slow any bleeding. Sometimes the area affected (hand, arm, foot or leg) will be immersed in cold water, or ice may be applied. The ice can surround the joint in the case of treatment for a sprain or it might be applied by rubbing a pulled muscle with an ice cup: a paper cup of water frozen in a freezer; as the ice melts the paper of the cup is torn away exposing more ice.

Initial treatment is summarized in the acronym PRICE-MM which stands for Protection, Rest, Ice, Compression, Elevation then Medications and Modalities. Most injuries require this PRICE treatment, which is designed to reduce further injury and to keep swelling down. Pain may also be reduced by using Medications: particularly non-steroidal anti-inflammatory drugs (NSAIDs). When tissue such as bone or muscle is injured, prostaglandins are released and they cause pain. Aspirin and related drugs are examples of NSAIDs that block the actions of the prostaglandins and reduce pain. However, the prostaglandins are released for a purpose, they aid tissue repair, so the pain relievers should be used only for as long as necessary.

Healing the injury generally requires additional treatment (using varying Modalities). After a few days, when bleeding has stopped, heat may be applied to stimulate blood flow and aid the healing process. Exercises, for both strength and flexibility, can aid in the recovery and in preventing the loss of necessary strength or flexibility during the healing process. Proper stretching can also reduce the formation of some scar tissue, which might otherwise tighten a muscle. But if the injury is to the muscle fibre stretching might increase the injury. Let the doctor decide.

Phases of Standard Treatment

What follows are descriptions of standard treatment of injuries commonly used by those who treat athletic injuries professionally. PRICE treatment is primary, and in many cases is the only treatment needed. Often, however, the injury is healed more quickly if the MM phase of treatment is applied at the right time. Heat or electrical stimulation, for instance, may be added to the treatment later in the rehabilitation process. The application of heat must be carefully timed: it can increase the blood flow to the damaged area, which brings needed nutrients such as calcium to a broken bone, but heat can increase swelling and it is safer to limit treatment to application of cold.

The standard treatment will help:

- pulled muscles
- twisted knees
- twisted or sprained ankles
- elbow problems
- shoulder injuries
- low back pain due to injury.

It will not affect a broken arm. No matter how much heat is applied, the injury will not heal any sooner than four to six weeks.

A well-conditioned player can move more quickly through the phases described, because with a more efficient circulatory system enzymes and nutrients are brought to the injury quickly and continuously. Often heat may be started almost immediately, possibly within a day. On the other hand, a less fit player will have to go through the phases as three-day periods.

Phase One: the first three days

The goal here is to stop and reduce swelling. The body usually reduces the swelling before it begins to heal the injury area. If there is a lot of swelling, the body will take longer to begin the healing process. The goal is to stop the swelling as much as possible before adding the heat which will help to heal the injury.

Use ice on the injured area for twenty minutes every two hours. It is better to enclose the whole injured area completely. A sprained ankle could be put into a bucket filled with ice water; a knee would need a larger enclosure, such as a bath tub. The water should be between 55° and 60° Fahrenheit (13–15° Celsius). The very cold water will reduce the blood circulation and thereby reduce swelling and scarring. The amount of time that each body part may need the ice may vary. For example, it is effective to ice a knee for five minutes, but twenty-five minutes is four times more effective in decreasing the blood flow to the knee.

If necessary, continue this two-hourly treatment for three days. If, after a day, the swelling has gone down, or remains the same, the next step is to begin heat, which promotes healing. If the swelling is stopped in the first three days, continuing to apply cold to the area is acceptable but it delays the opportunity to begin healing by the proper use of heat.

Phase Two: the second three days

This period is used both to reduce swelling and to promote healing. If the swelling has definitely stopped some heat can be applied, always followed by cold.

The standard treatment in phase two is: one minute warm, three minutes cold, alternating five times. End with five minutes of ice, to shut down any blood vessels that may have opened because of the heat and begun bleeding again. It is best to submerge the injured area in warm water but hot packs can also be used. While the injured area is in the warm water, the blood vessels are opening, bringing all the nutrients and enzymes into the area and beginning the healing process. Heat should be about 105–110° F (41–44°C). It should not be applied for too long a period of time.

Phase Three: the third three days

This period sees increased healing by more use of heat. During this period subtract one minute from the cold water time and add that minute to the warm water, so there will be two minutes in the warm water and two minutes in the cold. Alternate this treatment five times, ending with five minutes of cold to contract the blood vessels that are still not completely healed.

This should be done two to five times a day, if possible. With a full daily schedule it may be necessary to make a few adjustments in order to maximize the healing process. An example would be to get up a half hour earlier in the morning. The injury could be treated once before going out for the day, whether it be to work, school or college. If there is a break during the morning have another treatment. It may be convenient to use hot packs, which can be heated in a small pan of water, and cold packs, which might be ice cubes or a pack that can be put in the freezer.

Lunch break brings another opportunity for treatment. Repeat treatment at the end of the day and before you begin your exercise programme. If you exercise, do not repeat the treatment immediately after the practice. Rather, use ice or cold water to reduce any swelling that results. The last treatment will be just before bedtime.

This schedule would give you five treatments even during a busy day. But remember, the more times the warm and cold treatment is done over these three days, the more the healing process is accelerated.

Phase Four: the fourth three days

By the tenth day, the treatment becomes three minutes warm, one minute cold, alternating five times, ending with five minutes of cold. Use this routine five times a day. At the end of phase four, which is twelve days, the treatment is ten minutes of heat four to five times a day. Do not try to accelerate the treatment by using heat for more than ten minutes because more problems, such as unwanted swelling, are more likely.

If there is any swelling in the injury site go back to phase three treatment: cut down on the heat and add more cold to control the swelling. If necessary, go all the way back to phase two, and work back up again. After twenty-four days the injured site should be nearly back to normal.

Exercise during standard treatment

Exercise acts as additional therapy during the treatment process. Exercises should be begun as soon as possible after the injury, because the exercise helps reduce the formation of scar tissue.

The time to exercise the injured area, particularly a joint, is when it is being iced.

135

Because the ice is making the blood vessels contract, the swelling can be controlled. In the case of a sprained ankle, for instance, check the range of motion, to see how far the ankle can move in every direction. Take the ball of the foot and press the foot upward. Then move it downward. Then move the foot inward so that the sole of the foot is facing toward the other foot (inversion). Then roll the foot outward so that the sole is facing away from the other foot (eversion).

During phase one do these movements ten times during the icing phase of treatment. In phase two, while the injury is having three minutes of ice, do a great deal of movement of the joint.

Protecting the Injury

Protecting an injured area is important if you plan to continue playing soccer while the injury heals. A soft tissue injury, such as to the skin or muscles, is protected with a dough-nut-shaped pad to keep the pressure off of the injury and distribute it to the surrounding tissue. For a small blister perhaps a few thick-nesses of gauze pads will do, while to protect a larger area a thick felt or heavy sponge rubber 'doughnut' will work. Athletic training sup-pliers, pharmacies and many sporting goods stores usually have round or oval pads specifi-cally made for such protection. This will then be covered with a thicker pad that protects the injury and directs any pressure to the underly-ing pad. Protected in this way the injury will not be further irritated.

Athletic training tape can often be used to protect an injured joint or muscle. It may be used to limit the action of a joint, such as when taping an ankle or wrist, or it can be used completely to immobilize a joint, such as a finger or thumb. Certified athletic trainers are employed by most universities in the USA. Physical therapists are also generally adept at taping and are readily available in private practice.

FINDING THE BEST PROFESSIONAL TREATMENT

Consulting a good sports medicine medical doctor is generally the best option for effec-tive treatment. Not all doctors understand the most effective ways to get you back on the field quickly. For back injuries an effective chi-ropractor will often work wonders. It is gen-erally best, however, if a chiropractor works with a sports medicine specialist. Sometimes podiatrists can help with soccer-related foot problems. For pain, acupuncture from a skilled therapist often works. A number of medical doctors have taken special training in acupunc-ture. Magnet therapy also often works, espe-cially to speed the healing of fractures.

PSYCHOLOGICAL FACTORS IN INJURY AND RECOVERY

Two studies, both from the end of the last century, cast interesting light on the way the mind affects physical states. An Australian study (Andersen and Williams, 1999) measured the anxiety of college athletes and their visual changes and reaction times during stress. The subjects were also evaluated according to their life events, and their stresses from them, as well as their social support. The major finding was that the major predictor of future injury was the negative stress from their lives outside of sport.

In an American study on pain beliefs, it was found that there was no difference in most beliefs about pain, such as why it occurs or whether the athlete is to blame for the injury and pain. However, one significant finding was that the difference between the non-injured athletes and those who were severely injured was in their belief relative to how long the pain would last. While most of the athletes believed that the pain from an injury would be short-lived, those who were not injured believed that any pain from an injury would be very short. The athletes seemed to have believed that they were, to a large degree, in control of their own pain (O'Connor, 1991).

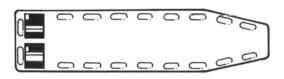

Brittany spine board with head stabilizer.

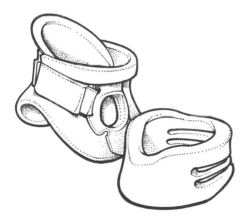

Cervical collars.

First aid supplies and equipment

To treat wounds

- 1½ inch athletic tape
- sterile pads
- non-stick pads
- gauze bandages: 1", 2", 4"
- sterile gloves
- antiseptic spray
- cleaning pads

To treat swelling

- ice
- instant cold packs
- freeze spray
- elastic wraps: 2", 4", 6"
- elastic tape

To immobilize breaks and sprains

- splints (air, formable aluminium, wood)
- cervical collar
- spinal board

To aid resuscitation

- airways (oropharyngeal and nasopharyngeal)
- Ambu bag
- oxygen
- defibrillator
- For suction
  'Venflon' or similar for cricothyroid or tension pneumothorax puncture
- For transportation
  stretcher; electric cart

PREPARATION FOR THE POSSIBILITIES OF INJURY

As with any other sport, the pitch-side medical team must have all the equipment and material that they may need.

Apart from the supplies and equipment listed in the box, there is the need for well-trained personnel. These personnel should be familiar with all the equipment, so that resuscitation and stabilization of any injury can be carried out efficiently and safely.

If medical personnel are not available for training or for a match someone trained in first aid should be available. More and more people involved in sports as coaches or trainers are being required to be certified in first aid techniques. A person with such training can reduce the chances of permanent harm from the injury, increase the chance of an earlier return of the athlete to action, and in some cases prevent a player's death.

Having said all this, there are thousands, if not millions, of games played every week without this type of support. Life-threatening injuries have not been reported routinely, so one might conclude that this type of injury is not that common. In élite soccer, resources are less of a problem. In minor league soccer, the equipment and personnel are often not available for financial reasons. However, like all insurance policies, risk assessment governs, and because of the relatively low incidence of serious injury in soccer, the expenditure is often deemed unnecessary.

From a professional point of view, if you are medically qualified, and providing medical cover for a game, you should make sure you have all the equipment and be adequately trained, as without either of these, you may leave yourself liable to litigation should anything untoward occur.

Standard treatment for any injury except a fracture

First three days: icing for 20 minutes every 2 hours (Begin manipulating an unjured joint during the cold treatment)

Second three days: 1 minute warm, 3 minutes cold

Third three days: 2 minutes warm, 2 minutes cold

Fourth three days: 3 minutes warm, 1 minute cold

Stretch and strengthen the affected area continually

CHAPTER 14

Injuries to the Head and Neck

HEAD INJURY

When we talk about head injury, we generally mean brain injury, or concussion. There are often, of course, associated soft tissue and bony injuries. Head injuries are common in soccer. Studies find the incidence to be about 12%, with 20% of those head injuries to be concussions.

Causes of Head Injury

Heading the ball is an integral part of the game, and there has been some concern over the years about how much accumulative damage is done to the brain by heading. Some players head the ball much more than others. Some central defenders and strikers are famous for aerial power, and hence will

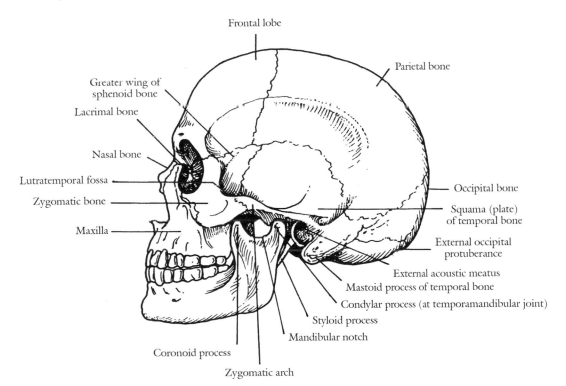

The skull.

Frontal lobe

Parietal bone

Greater wing of
sphenoid bone

Lacrimal bone

Nasal bone

Lutratemporal fossa

Zygomatic bone

Maxilla

Occipital bone

Squama (plate)
of temporal bone

External occipital
protuberance

External acoustic meatus

Mastoid process of temporal bone

Condylar process (at temporamandibular joint)

Styloid process

Mandibular notch

Coronoid process

Zygomatic arch

head the ball more, both in practice and in games. In years past, balls were much heavier, and even more so when wet. Now, balls are coated with waterproofing, and their weight is more constant despite the prevailing weather. Having said this, balls travel much faster now so more brain trauma may be possible.

The debate about occupational injury in soccer will rage on, and head injury will be part of it. Apart from all this, there are head injuries that are not a result of heading the ball, but from trauma. A clash of heads ('head banging') when two players challenge to head the ball at the same time is the most common. Occasionally, players get kicked in the head, and, of course, foul play can result in head injury.

Any player with dizziness, headache or neck pain after heading a ball should be evaluated for a mild concussion. Usually this just requires removing the player from the game, but repeated complaints need to be seriously considered for medical evaluation.

Diagnosis

The diagnosis of head injury is straightforward, inasmuch as head trauma is overt, and players, or others on the field of play, know that a head injury has occurred. The diagnosis lies in the extent of the concussion, and this is where the difficulty starts. When entering the field of play to assess the extent of injury, the trainer, physiotherapist or doctor has only one decision to make: can the player continue or not?

Initial assessment

Is the player conscious? If not, first aid, following the normal ABC protocol (airway, breathing, circulation) should be employed. If the player is breathing but unconscious, the airway must be protected. This may be done by putting the player in the recovery position. Before this, however, care should be taken if there is a possibility of a coexisting neck injury. If this is so, the airway can be protected by the use of oro-pharyngeal or naso-pharyngeal airways. The neck must then be protected by the use of in-line cervical immobilization, with the use of a collar and a spinal board. The player should then be safely removed from the field of play for further assessment.

In most cases, however, the player with a head injury is conscious with no other associated injury, and this makes harder the decision about continuing to play.

It is necessary to evaluate four memory factors, with the acronym COID:

1 **C**oncentration
2 **O**rientation
3 **I**mmediate memory, and
4 **D**elayed recall.

A quick check can be undertaken using 'Maddock's questions':

- Immediate memory: immediate recall of three words
- Delayed recall: recall of three words after fifteen minutes
- Recent memory: 'What's the score?' 'Which half is the game in, first or second?' 'Who scored last?' 'Which way are you playing'
- Concentration: Serial sevens and threes.

Supplementary questions may be asked, for instance 'What was the score last week?'

There are difficulties in all this. Often, the player just wants to go on playing. Sometimes the questions are answered, but not always as adequately as they could be. The real problem is that there are no reliable tests for the extent of a concussion that can be used on the field of play. Maddock's questions give us a good guess, but they are by no means definitive, and are therefore subject to potential pitfalls in interpretation. If the player exits play, further evaluation must take place, and hospitalization arranged if it is believed to be necessary. If the player continues to play, this evaluation should take place at the end of the match.

In a way, the more difficult decision comes after the match. When can a player return to train and play? The debate around this is based upon the fact that there is no easy way to determine the extent of injury to the brain. In rugby union, if a player is concussed, he is out for three weeks. How does one measure concussion? Well, there is no grading of concussion, and the severity really depends on the COID, Maddock's questions, and formal psychometric testing.

Psychometric testing

This method examines brain function rather than anatomy. In brain injury or concussion, function is impaired and this can be measured. However, to do this effectively, players must be assessed before injury, as it is the change in psychometric measurements that is important. In the section of this book about screening (Chapter 4), psychometric testing was mentioned. There are now web-based tests that are easy to access, but they are somewhat expensive. The digital symbol substitution test (DSST) is available in many textbooks, and although not as sensitive as the web-based tests, it is cheap and easy to administer: no computer is needed.

If psychometric testing is carried out as part of the screening process when a player joins a team, or at the beginning of a season, this gives the medical team a chance to rehabilitate the player from head injury safely. Serial measurements can be made after a head injury, and return to train and play can be carefully managed. From a litigation point of view, it may be that in the future, clubs and teams may be liable if it cannot be shown that return to play after a head injury was appropriately managed.

Brain imaging

If the trauma is severe, brain swelling or contusion may be seen when performing MRI or CT scans. However, with a mild to moderate concussion, changes are usually absent, so this can lead to a false sense of security. It is easy to let the player back onto the team, especially if there is pressure from the player or coach or both.

Extra-dural Haemorrhage

The dura mater is a strong fibrous 'bag' surrounding the brain and spinal cord. It lies between the brain and the inside of the skull. Inside the bag is the cerebro-spinal fluid (CSF), which bathes the brain and spinal cord. Hence there is a fluid cushion enclosed in the dura mater that helps to protect the brain. Extra-dural haemorrhage is a serious type of head injury that can happen at any age, but more often in young people.

This injury occurs when there is trauma to the area of the side of the head known as the temple. In this area there is an artery that goes through the skull. If the trauma is sufficiently forceful, this artery fractures. The blood can then collect in the area between the dura mater and the skull. The blood causes compression on the brain, and can eventually lead to death if not treated. The treatment is to remove the blood surgically. Full recovery can be expected if treated promptly.

Specific Injuries

Severe cuts

These can bleed as if the player is about to exsanguinate: to be drained of blood. It can be an emotional experience if other players, officials or spectators see lots of blood. The job of the medical personnel at a match is to stem the bleeding as quickly as possible. This is done by simple direct pressure over the wound. Sterile gloves should be worn. Surgical gauze is a good material to use for pressure. The player may need to leave the field whilst the blood flow is stemmed, and the cut may require glue, steri-strips, stitches or all three. The cut must be cleaned first, and all foreign matter removed.

If the player needs to continue, there are coagulation sprays which will quickly stop the bleeding. If the wound can be occluded with a dressing or bandage, the player may be able to carry on. The referee will decide whether continuing is safe. Some sports do not allow a return to the match if there is blood because of the possibility of blood-borne infection such as HIV. The player may need to change clothes if they are bloody. If the player does continue, appropriate closure can be obtained after the match is over. There are regions on the face that may require specialist suturing techniques. Around the eye, and across the line of the lip are areas that can be problematic if not sutured properly.

Zygoma fracture

Because of its location, just below the eye, the cheek-bone, or zygoma, is prone to injury. It gets injured by sustaining a direct kick, by being 'headed' in an aerial challenge, and by the foul use of the elbow. The appearance of the cheekbone is flattened, although this may not be obvious due to swelling. There is often a 'step' felt as the examiner runs their finger along the bone. The treatment is surgical, and the bone is repositioned. There will be an associated concussion, which should not be forgotten. The injury takes approximately four weeks to recover from.

Orbital fracture

This is a fracture around the eye socket. It is sustained in a similar way to the zygoma fracture. Observation will show that there is obvious swelling, though bruising may not be evident just after an injury. The eyeball appears recessed, and there is a loss of sensation just below the eye, due to pressure on the nerve supplying that area, which runs in the floor of the eye socket. The player will complain of double vision. Treatment is prompt surgical intervention, and the timing of return to play will depend on the extent of the injury.

Tooth fracture or avulsion (loss of tooth)

Teeth are important for a player's appearance as well as the need to chew food. If an injured player has a tooth (or teeth) missing, check that the airway is clear. Loose teeth or bits of tooth are easily caught in the trachea and can cause respiratory obstruction.

A tooth injury needs effective emergency management as this will result in the best outcome. It may be possible to restore a broken or dislodged tooth, so if possible the player should keep it in the mouth, between cheek and gum. If that is not possible, it should be wrapped in silver paper and bathed in milk. An urgent opinion from a dentist should be sought, as the true extent of the injury needs to be assessed.

Nasal injuries

These are common. It may be necessary to arrange an X-ray to delineate the injury, and possibly referral to an Ear, Nose and Throat (ENT) specialist for surgical intervention. In professional soccer, players will wait until a convenient time, either the close of the season or end of their career, before consenting to surgery. However, if the airway is not open, intervention may be needed sooner rather than later. The attending physician should assess the airways, and make sure that there is no sub-mucous haematoma over the nasal cartilage. If this is the case, the mucosa cannot nourish the cartilage, and it dies, leaving the player with a flattened nose. The haematoma, if recognized, should be drained as soon as possible.

Eye injuries

These are not common in soccer, but are obviously important when they do occur. Corneal abrasions can be very painful, and are usually caused by the accidental poking of a finger in the eye. They can be seen by putting fluoroscein drops in the eye, and then shining a blue filter light diagonally at the eye. A line of fluoroscein can be seen where the abrasion is. It should be treated with local anaesthetic drops (benoxinate or amethocaine) then the eye should be covered. Local anaesthetic drops should not be used unless the eye will be covered, as the blink reflex to dust or trauma will be dulled, and further damage may ensue. Drops to dilate the pupil (e.g. tropicamide) sometimes help with the pain.

Trauma to the eye can cause more serious problems. Vitreous haemorrhage can occur. The vitreous humour is a protective cushion in the eye that lies in the eye itself, between the back and the front of the eyeball. Vitreous haemorrhage is diagnosed if a light is shone into the eye. Instead of the normal red colour being reflected back, there is no reflection. Comparison should be made with the other eye. Occasionally, the trauma can be severe enough to cause swelling of the retina. The retina is at the back of the eye where the sight-sensing nerves are. Swelling around here stops the nerves from working properly, and the player gets blurred vision. This can be dangerous if the eye sustains further trauma, as this can lead to retinal detachment. The treatment for both of these is rest, although retinal detachment may require laser treatment, but expert opinion from an ophthalmologist should be sought. The real problem with the eye is that it often appears quiet on the surface, but can be badly injured underneath, so be vigilant.

NECK INJURY

The neck is exposed to injury for two main reasons. Firstly, the neck is equivalent to a

143

piece of string connecting two large medicine balls, of differing weight. It is easy to imagine what happens to the 'string' if the analogous medicine balls are thrown. It gets stretched, pulled around and sometimes broken. The second point is that the musculature in the neck is often unable to resist these forces.

In soccer, thankfully, the incidence of neck injury is relatively uncommon. These injuries often occur at the same time as a head injury, and can easily be overlooked. In fact, if a player sustains a head injury, there is a neck injury too. It is just a question of severity. If the spinal cord is injured at the neck, paralysis, and sometimes death, can occur.

The neck is hard to examine on the field of play. The decision about how to treat such an injury is largely based on the observation of the pitch-side medical team, and the history given by the player. The most important point is that if there is any doubt, then use in-line spinal mobilization with a collar. If the player

proves to have a trivial injury, it may look as if you over-reacted. However, much better this than believing the injury to be a trivial one, and it proving much worse.

Whiplash

This is an injury of the neck that is caused by sudden, forced and uncontrolled extension (bending backwards) or flexion (bending forwards) of the neck, or both. The injury can involve any or all of the structures in the neck. The whiplash syndrome often develops into a chronic problem because of scarring in the ligaments around the spine, and damage to the small joints that help hold the spine together.

Although usually associated with road traffic accidents, being shoved and bumped when jumping for a ball exerts similar forces on the neck. Most of this type of injury incurred in soccer is of a minor type. Players who habitually head the ball will suffer some degree of this during most matches, and in

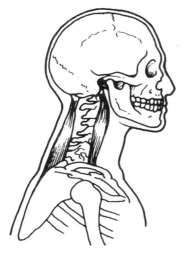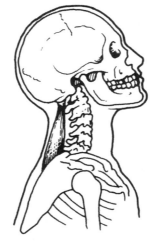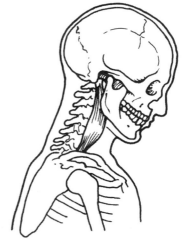

The muscles of the neck.

training. The more severe cases are treated symptomatically, but if there is a neurological deficit of any kind (for instance weakness, numbness or pins and needles), referral should be made so that the injury can be investigated fully before allowing a return to play. Although whiplash is common, it can be part of a more extensive injury to the neck, which needs clarification, and treatment.

Facet joint strain

The facet joints are small joints that sit between each vertebra, aiding stability. They are located just behind, and to the side of, the channel where the spinal cord runs. Structurally, they are similar to the shoulder, hip, and knee joints. The two bony halves of the joint are lined by hyaline cartilage (see Chapter 3), the smooth membrane that helps re-distribute the forces in the joint experienced during movement. The joints are enveloped in a capsule. These joints are injured in forced extension of the neck, when they are jammed together, and in uncontrolled rotation of the neck, when one or other of the joints are jammed together. Disruption can cause severe pain, with restriction of movement, and even nerve symptoms down the arm. The joints are situated near where the nerve comes out of the spine, and any swelling can cause local pressure on the nerve.

When a facet joint strain first happens, it may be part of a serious neck injury. If so, then appropriate first aid measures, with cervical collar and immobilization should be used. The player should be carefully assessed in the medical room, and if there is any doubt, be sent to a hospital for fuller examination.

Better to be over-cautious than have a player who ends up paralysed.

Disc damage

The spine is made up of twenty-four vertebrae, each separated by a disc. The discs are a bit like ring doughnuts, with thick jam in the middle. The outer rim is a strong gristle-like substance that maintains the distance between each vertebra. The middle (like jam) acts to distribute pressure around the disc during movement. This is a good system for the type of movements needed during everyday activity, but forced movements can cause disruption of the outer rim of the disc. This can happen to varying degrees, but if the rim is breached, the jam-like centre can escape. If it escapes it usually ends up opposite the facet joint. This is a slipped disc, and if there is enough of the 'jam', there will be pressure on the nerve as it comes out of the spine. This causes pain, numbness, and pins and needles in the arm. Once again, the extent of the injury can be difficult to measure pitchside. If there is any doubt, the treatment is immobilization, removal, and hospitalization (if necessary).

Fractures

There is a recognized system of classification of fractures, which is beyond the scope of this book. However, the mechanism of injury is very similar to that previously mentioned for other neck injuries. Whilst it may be that more force is required to achieve fracture, this may not be the case; it is how the forces are distributed that decide when the bone 'gives way', resulting in a fracture. The on-field management is the same.

145

CHAPTER 15

Injuries to the Thorax, Chest and Shoulders

From a practical point of view, the chest and the thorax are more or less the same. It consists of a cage of ribs, with a bone in the front, the sternum or breastbone, and the spine at the back. The ribs attach to the spine by way of two small joints. If you have ever seen a piece of meat from the area around the spine of an animal, you will be able to see where the ribs join the spine. The ribs attach to the breastbone via a small rib-shaped piece of cartilage. This enables the chest to expand and contract whilst breathing; without it, the rib cage would be rigid. The cage is there to protect the vital organs it encloses: the heart, the lungs, the liver, and the large blood vessels feeding these. As soon as the anatomy is evident, and knowing football, it is clear how injuries occur.

DIRECT BLOWS TO THE CHEST

Rib Injuries

The most common chest injury is a cracked, or fractured, rib. A collision is usually the cause. They can be very painful, as the chest, and hence the fracture, will move with every breath. In the early stages of this injury, the player will not let anyone get near for fear of the lightest nudge, or worse, that someone

will make them laugh, which is agony. Occasionally when a rib fractures, the two ends of the bones may be displaced. In this case, the sharp end of the rib can puncture the lung and cause a collapsed lung, or pneumothorax. This causes shortness of breath. Difficulty in diagnosis arises because the player cannot breathe properly anyway because of the pain, which gives the impression of being short of ('out of') breath.

In any event, it is usual for the player to have to leave the field, and a more thorough examination can take place in the medical room. If there is any doubt, the player should be sent to a hospital for an X-ray examination. In extensive cases, a tube may be put into the chest cavity to 'drain' the air that has escaped

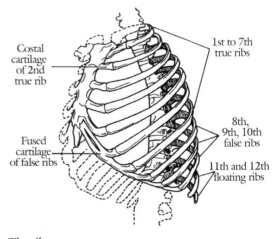

Costal cartilage of 2nd true rib

1st to 7th true ribs

8th, 9th, 10th false ribs

Fused cartilage of false ribs

11th and 12th floating ribs

The ribs.

146

from the lung puncture. In so doing, the collapsed lung re-inflates.

The most unusual type of rib injury is one where the rib comes through the skin. In this instance, a valve effect can be set up where air is drawn into the lung cavity, causing a build-up of pressure in the chest. This build-up can eventually stop air and blood entering the lungs and heart respectively, with catastrophic consequences. Again, shortness of breath is the predominant symptom. Prompt action by inserting a needle into the affected side of the chest relieves the pressure, and recovery is usually spectacular.

Fractured ribs have often been treated with strapping to prevent excessive movement, but nothing has ever been shown to help. They take about six weeks to heal, and although the player may practise and train before this, he may not be able to enter into contact until this period is over. The coach or manager should be made aware of this fact so they can plan the return to play appropriately.

In younger athletes especially, the ribs and chest wall go out of shape much more easily in response to pressure or trauma than in adults. In the very unusual syndrome sudden death can be the result of a blow to the chest. If sufficiently strong, this blow causes the heart to dysfunction. Similar blows can cause rupture of the main blood vessels in the chest. These occurrences, though tragic, are very rare.

Sternum Bruise

In soccer, the breastbone is often bruised, but hardly ever seriously. It can be painful, especially when breathing, coughing or sneezing. The central origin of the pain may give rise to concern that the pain is of cardiac origin. By pressing on the sternum and reproducing the pain, you can confirm why the pain is there.

Occasionally, and always from major trauma, the breastbone can be fractured. This is very painful, and causes severe bruising over the ensuing weeks, before full recovery at six weeks. If this is suspected it is reasonable to order an X-ray. There is no active treatment, except painkillers. A complication, however, is that because of the pain, the player's breathing may be more shallow than normal, and coughing is far too painful. The normal function of coughing and clearing the throat is to clear the lungs of breathed-in debris. This debris is normally carried to the top of the lungs by small hairs, called cilia, that move the matter upwards until it arrives at the back of the throat where it is coughed up, then swallowed. If this process is not continuously carried out the debris, and associated mucous, lies in the lungs and can easily become infected, making the whole thing worse, as a chest infection will cause even more coughing. Hence, the use of adequate painkillers for this and for fractured or bruised ribs is important, as it aids normal function.

SHOULDER INJURIES

Shoulder injuries are, for obvious reasons, less common in soccer players. The exception to this is goalkeepers.

Dislocated Shoulder

A shoulder dislocation occurs when the 'ball' of the joint leaves its 'socket'. This commonly happens when a player tries to break a fall by sticking an arm out. Whether one lands on the hand, with a stiff arm, or on the elbow, the

147

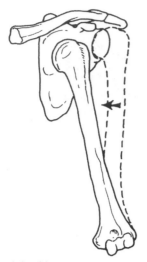

A dislocated shoulder.

force of the blow is transferred to the weakest part of the whole appendage and the weakest part goes. This might be a bone breaking or an elbow dislocating, but is more commonly the shoulder joint dislodging.

The shoulder is a specialized joint. It has great mobility, but pays for this with a lack of stability. The ball, which is at the top of the humerus (the bone in the upper arm), has a very spherical shape, but the socket is quite shallow. It has a rim of cartilage around the edge that helps stability, but in the traumatic situations that arise in soccer this is not enough to prevent dislocation. In over 90% of cases, the socket dislocates forwards and downwards. This causes pain, and may be associated with a fracture to the humerus itself.

In dislocation, the rim of cartilage mentioned above gets brushed off, sometimes with a chip of bone. This can cause recurrent dislocation if not treated, and requires surgery. There is a nerve that runs around the narrowing of the humerus just below the top, where the ball is, called the axillary nerve. This can

get caught up in the tissues during the trauma of dislocation and cause permanent damage. This nerve activates the deltoid muscle, which is the large muscle at the top of the arm. If the nerve is damaged, the muscle will not work properly, and although recovery may take place, it may be months before it happens, and recovery may not be complete.

There has been debate over the years about the emergency treatment of shoulder dislocation. The current recommendation is that the player should be removed from the field of play and X-rayed. The shoulder can then only be reduced (humerus put back into the shoulder socket) once a fracture has been ruled out. After reduction, a period of enforced rest is necessary to allow the joint capsule and surrounding tissues to heal. This takes about six weeks, after which a period of rehabilitation is undertaken. This takes the form of strengthening the stabilizing muscles around the shoulder (*see* Chapter 12), and endeavouring to regain normal function. The player will then return to play step by step, with training first, then half a game, then a full game.

Occasionally the shoulder, although apparently back to normal, dislocates again, this time with much less force than that which caused the original injury. This is a worrying event, as it may mean that the restraining structures around the joint (the rim of cartilage for instance) are damaged, and cannot perform their functions properly. If this is the case, the player may need to consult a specialist shoulder surgeon, with a view to surgical stabilization. Although rehabilitation will successfully aid return to play after surgery, this obviously takes a longer time, usually three months. There are commercially made harnesses that reduce the chance of re-injuring the joint.

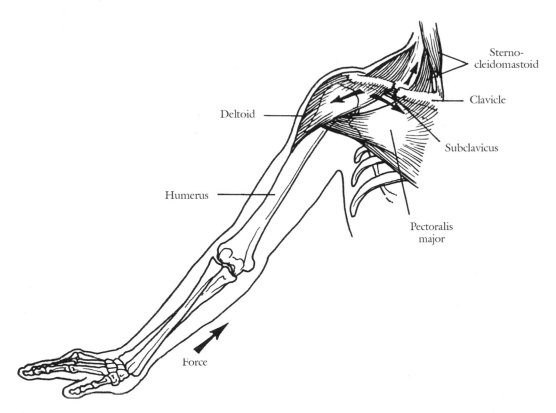

Sterno-
cleidomastoid

Clavicle

Deltoid

Subclavicus

Humerus

Pectoralis
major

Force

A fractured collarbone.

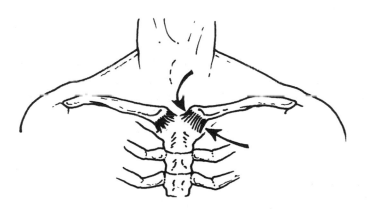

Sprained ligament at collarbone–sternum joint.

149

Posterior dislocation, although uncommon, can occur, and should be treated in exactly the same way. Recurrence is less common, however, due to the restraining structures at the back of the shoulder.

Acromio–clavicular Joint Disruption

The shoulder blade sits at the back of the chest. There is a part of the scapula, called the acromion, that runs forwards and outwards, and arrives above the shoulder joint. Here it meets the collarbone, or clavicle. This joint is called the acromio–clavicular joint. It consists of two flat parts of each bone that meet, and are bound together by strong ligaments. There are also two strong ligaments that tie the end of the collarbone down to the top of the main part of the shoulder blade.

During soccer play, there are many instances of shoulders coming together in challenges for the ball. Falling sideways on the edge of the shoulder is also common. Both these occur often in goalkeepers. When this happens with sufficient force, the joint tends to separate. In this situation, the ligaments are not strong enough to hold it together. There are different grades of this injury, from a mild sprain with some discomfort, to complete dislocation, with severe pain.

Treatment is usually non-surgical. An X-ray will confirm that there is no associated fracture. Pain relief, including anti-inflamma-

tories will help. There may be a lot of bruising depending on the degree of injury. Taping to try to depress the collarbone back into position can help the pain, and may reduce the amount of residual deformity. This deformity is a lump on the top of the shoulder joint. Although not unsightly, it can make an asymmetry that may cause concern. Surgery has been undertaken for this injury, but this restricts the natural movement of the bones in this area, and has largely been discontinued except for the most extreme cases.

Fractured Clavicle

This is usually caused by falling on an outstretched arm. The force of the fall is transmitted up the arm, across the shoulder joint, to the clavicle, which breaks. This is usually at the junction between the outer and middle thirds of the bone. Occasionally, direct trauma, perhaps from another player's fall, can cause a fracture. The player feels immediate pain, and when assessed on the field, a step can sometimes be felt along the bone, at the point of maximal tenderness. The step is not always evident, but what is evident is that the player cannot carry on. X-ray examination reveals the fracture, and most will heal with a collar and cuff support, which takes about six weeks.

Occasionally, the bone does not heal so easily, especially if there are multiple fragments, and may need surgical fixation.

CHAPTER 16

Injuries to the Arms and Hands

ARM INJURIES

Fractures of the Humerus

It is useful to split these into those fractures around the part of the humerus near the top (proximal), and those near the bottom (distal).

The position of fracture of the humerus is important because of the structures around the bone. Fractures of different places in the humerus can cause injury to the nerves and blood vessels that travel down the arm. This damage can be very serious if not noticed and treated.

The part of the humerus just below the top, where it forms half of the shoulder joint, is called the neck. The part of this bone that is in the joint itself is called, logically, the head. Fractures of the neck of the humerus are caused by direct trauma to the arm in a fall

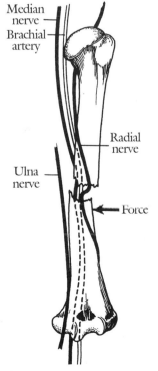

Humerus fracture.

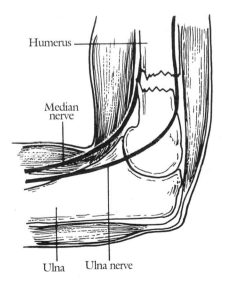

Lower humerus fracture.

or by a kick, or by falling on an outstretched arm. There is immediate pain and the player is unable to carry on playing. On examination, there may be some swelling, and tenderness in the arm. When standing, the player may try to support the injured arm with the other hand. This is not an uncommon observation in arm, shoulder, and collarbone injuries. The mechanism of injury will give you a guide to the diagnosis.

The player should be X-rayed, and if it is a fracture, a collar and cuff is applied. In the soccer-playing population, that is to say, the active not-old, these fractures take approximately six weeks to heal. With immobilization, the shoulder joint can become stiff and itself require rehabilitation. This may prolong the time to return to play, and of course, this has greater significance in goalkeepers, who will have lost some of the muscular strength and control that goes with immobilization. Very occasionally, the bone fails to heal and may need surgical fixation.

Supracondylar Fracture

This is a fracture of the humerus just above the elbow. The 'condyles' are the small prominences felt either side of the elbow, so this fracture is superior to (above) these condyles. It is more common in the young, but can occur at any age.

When a bone is fractured, the muscles that usually act in concert to move a limb in the desired way start to contract. This is a reflex response to the pain. In this situation, the triceps muscle (which has its insertion at the back of the elbow, and straightens the elbow) goes into spasm, and pulls the point of the elbow backwards, and with it, the lower frag-

ment of the humerus. This leaves the blood vessels and nerves that run across the front of the joint exposed to the other fragment.

Always be vigilant for this type of fracture even though not all become displaced and potentially problematic. Examination may show that the back of the elbow sticks out more than normal. This is a sign that the fracture is displaced. Both forearm pulses should be sought. If they are absent this should be noted. The player should be sent to the hospital immediately for X-ray and expert opinion. Depending on the X-ray appearance, and whether the pulses in the forearm are present, the treatment may be plaster cast immobilization, or possibly surgical fixation. The complication of this type of injury can be forearm contracture if the blood supply is interrupted for too long, or loss of muscle action if the nerves are compromised.

Elbow Dislocation

This is unusual in football. It occurs when the player falls awkwardly. About 80% of the time, occurs when the bones of the forearm dislocate backwards out of the joint that they have with the humerus. The player, as would be expected, feels severe pain, and has to leave the field. Examination in skilled hands may be able to distinguish between a dislocation and a supracondylar fracture (see above), but this may be difficult due to pain, and swelling. Similarly, because of the structures that pass across the joint, an assessment of the pulses in the forearm should be made. Their absence or presence should be noted at first examination, and this information passed on to the hospital when attending for X-ray. The X-ray will confirm the diagnosis, and the bones can be replaced into the correct position (reduction). After reduction, the pulses should be re-assessed. If there has been a change from presence to absence, this is a reason to perform surgery, as it would appear that the trauma of relocation has obstructed the artery that is located in front of the joint. In rare situations an elbow dislocation occurs which is not associated with the degree of trauma necessary to cause the bones to poke out through the skin.

Recovery to full function may take six to eight weeks, and care must be taken, especially with goalkeepers, that a full range of motion is regained. Without care, the player may be left with a loss of extension (straightening) of the joint. In the throwing arm of a goalkeeper this could make the difference between being the best, and not.

Forearm Fractures

The two bones in the forearm are called the radius and the ulna. The radius runs down one side of the forearm, and ends just below the thumb. The ulna runs down the other side, and ends just below the small finger.

The two bones are joined by a strong fibrous band throughout most of their length. This is called the interosseus ('between bones') band. Both of these bones can be fractured. If a fracture is suspected, the player should obviously undergo X-ray examination. The X-rays must always include both ends of the bones in the forearm. Although a fracture in one of the bones may be obvious, there may be an occult (invisible) one in the other forearm bone.

The treatment depends on the type, and extent of the fracture(s). It may take the form of plaster cast immobilization, or surgical fixation. In these cases, expert orthopaedic opinion should be sought. The way that the bones work in unison can be spoiled, and the player may be left with forearm dysfunction. This often takes the form of a lack of rotation in the action of 'turning your hand over'. The most common fracture of the forearm seen in soccer is the colles fracture. This fracture involves the end of the radius (the bone that ends at the base of the thumb), and is caused by falling on an outstretched arm. It occurs commonly in elderly women suffering from osteoporosis. It is treated in accident and emergency by immobilization in a cast.

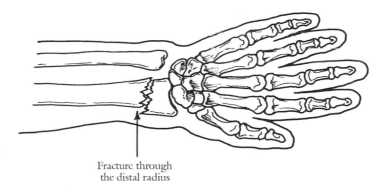

Fracture through
the distal radius

Wrist fracture (ulna).

153

WRIST AND HAND INJURIES

The wrist joint is formed between the radius and ulna, and the carpal bones. The joint is a specialized one that acts as a conduit to allow the extension of the arm to be effective in, for instance, obtaining food, or fending off predators, by efficient use of the hand.

From an injury point of view, there is a plate of cartilage, not unlike that in the shoulder and knee, that sits between the ulna and two of the carpal bones. This can become compressed in certain actions, especially throwing by goalkeepers. If the throwing technique can be altered, it may be that the compressive forces may be minimized. However, if this is not possible, the pain associated with this unusual injury may become constant, and severe enough to interfere with training and playing. In this case, anti-inflammatory tablets may be used. If not effective, local steroid injection can be given, but if pain persists, surgery may be necessary. This alters the mechanics of the wrist, and may promote degenerative change later in life. It also involves a long lay-off in terms of rehabilitation.

Scaphoid Fracture

The scaphoid is a carpal bone that forms the other side of the wrist joint by articulating with the radius. Scaphoid fracture is caused by falling on an outstretched hand and can be a real problem. The blood supply to the scaphoid is such that the main artery supplying the bone does not 'plug' itself in at the first available opportunity. It does so at the further part of the bone. This is fine unless the fall, and ensuing fracture, happens in the middle of the bone. This then cuts the blood

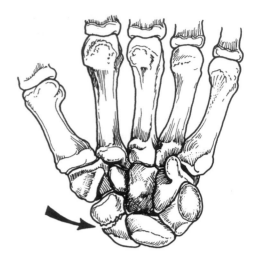

Scaphoid fracture.

supply off from the near end of the bone, and death of the bone can follow. This is compounded by the fact that initial X-ray of this area can look normal, in spite of the presence of a fracture.

The management of this type of injury is to start with an examination of an area called the 'anatomical snuff box'. This is situated on the edge of the wrist joint, between the top of the radius, and the scaphoid itself. If there is tenderness, the player should be sent for X-ray. If this is normal, and re-examination still shows tenderness, the forearm should be immobilized in a cast, and X-rayed again in seven to ten days time. Alternatively, and if access is possible, an isotope bone, CT, or MRI scan will unveil the diagnosis. Early recognition is essential to avoid a 'non-union', which is where the bone refuses to heal. Healing of any tissue requires blood supply, and early immobilization will give the best chance of maintaining that supply. However, there is no guarantee that early recognition and appropriate treatment will be effective, and failure to heal does happen. Surgical fixation, with bone grafting and growth factors can retrieve the situation, but occasionally a prosthesis (false bone) has to be inserted.

First Metacarpo-phalangeal Joint Ulnar Collateral Ligament Sprain

A long name for an injury to a small, but troublesome structure, this is sometimes called skier's thumb or gamekeeper's thumb. Like all collateral ligaments, this one sits between two bones, and these are found at the web between the thumb itself, and the index finger. If you put your finger in that web, then push onto the thumb, your finger will be on this ligament. It is called the ulnar collateral, because when standing upright in the anatomical position, with palms facing front, the ligament is on the ulnar side of the thumb, that is, nearer the middle.

This ligament is injured by falling forwards with the palm outstretched. The web mentioned above stretches, but then acts as a lever when the tip of the thumb hits the floor. The thumb bends outwards away from the index finger, spraining, tearing, or even rupturing the ligament. Occasionally, the ligament may pull off a small bony fragment which, if displaced, will need surgical fixation.

The diagnosis is evident, as stressing and pressing on the ligament causes pain. Swelling may occur, but if this is evident even on the field, there may well be a fracture. If a fracture is suspected, the player should leave the field, for fear of displacement of the fragment, and be X-rayed. If the ligament is sprained only, the thumb may be strapped to support the ligament. In a goalkeeper, this injury requires leaving the field as it may well impair function, especially if it involves the throwing hand.

Treatment is the PRICE regime, while decisions about the severity of the injury are made. If X-ray reveals a fracture, or suggests rupture, the thumb should be strapped, and a surgical opinion sought.

If the ligament is disrupted but not fractured, treatment focuses on aiding healing without leaving it loose, and this is done keeping the ligament short whilst in the healing phase. The use of taping will make sure that the best result is achieved. There is no guarantee that laxity will be avoided even if the correct treatment is administered. Even after rehabilitation, the ligament disruption can take varying amounts of time depending on the extent of fibre involvement. The discomfort in catching a ball, or even everyday things like unscrewing lids, can last for months, and protective taping may be required.

This injury can only be prevented by taping the thumb and index finger together, or at least closer. The difficulty is that taping may well interfere with function, and be unacceptable. As ever, it is up to the player to weigh the benefits and drawbacks of this type of intervention.

Metacarpal Fracture

This is an injury more commonly seen after a fight rather than in soccer. The metacarpal bones are the ones that join the carpal bones of the wrist to the fingers. They can easily be felt on the back of the hand as hard ridges. They are occasionally fractured in soccer by direct trauma, usually by kicking or being trodden upon. Often, during a game, there is pain inhibition, the fractures can be easily felt, and the fragments be moved without too much discomfort. Often a player will play the game and report the injury only after the game is ended. An X-ray will confirm the injury.

Most of the time, the injury heals itself if it has been immobilized in a cast or with taping. It should take four to six weeks. Occasionally, especially with the metacarpal associated with the small finger, there may be a displacement that needs surgical fixation.

Mallet Finger

To enable the fingers to move, there are tendons attached to various points on the back and the front of the bones of the fingers, called the phalanges (singular = phalanx). There are three phalanges in the fingers, two in the thumb. The last phalanx of the fingers has a tendon attached to it at the front and at the back. The tendon at the back can be pulled off, or avulsed, leaving the tip of the finger 'droopy'. This droopiness is caused by the action of the tendon on the front of the hand being intact, whilst the one at the back of the hand is absent. The deformity caused by this injury is called a mallet finger.

It is usually caused by direct trauma to the tip of the finger, which is forced into flexion (forcing the finger into the palm), thereby causing a stretching, then breaking, of the tendon. This deformity, although not serious, can interfere with daily life. For instance, putting your hands in a pocket can be problematic if a finger keeps getting caught on the outside of the pocket when the rest of your hand is inside.

The treatment is to wear a finger splint. The tendon eventually heals with a return to full function. This may take some months. Occasionally the finger fails to heal, and surgical repair can be attempted.

The use of a splint will protect an already, or previously, injured finger. However, the use of splints to protect would be impractical. Occasionally taping may suffice, but again, is impractical.

Return to normal function brings with it the strength and proprioception required for normal life. However, for goalkeepers specific exercises should be undertaken. These take the form of the use of sponge balls or old soft tennis balls to regain flexor strength, and extensor exercises for the finger involved. In normal life, the function returns without specific exercises, but in élite soccer it is important for players to return fully fit as soon as possible.

Taping the fingers in a spiral fashion can help prevent forced flexion. The drawback is that some flexibility will be lost. Players can try these measures, but firstly in training, never for the first time in a game.

CHAPTER 17
Injuries to the Spine

THE SPINE

The spine in the neck, or cervical spine, is covered in Chapter 14. In this chapter are

details of injuries to the thoracic and lumbar spines. The thoracic spine consists of the twelve vertebrae that have ribs attached to them. Although, as mentioned above, ribs do commonly get injured, the thoracic spine itself is seldom injured in soccer.

The lumbar spine is different, commonly being involved in complex injuries. It consists of the lower five vertebrae. The anatomy of the lumbar spine is exactly analogous to that of the cervical spine. There are some subtle differences, however. The body of each vertebra is larger, as more weight is borne by these in comparison with those in the neck. The small (facet) joints are at a slightly different angle than those in the neck. This allows movement in a different way, in line with environmental requirements.

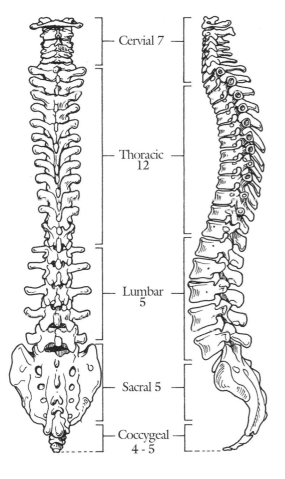

The spine.

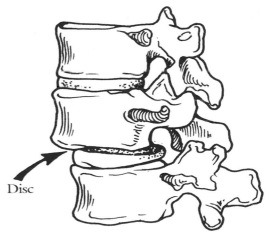

Vertebrae and discs.

Lumbar spine injuries are common in soccer, and relate to the anatomy of the spine, the stability of the pelvic and abdominal muscles, and the player's age. The issue of stability is covered later in this chapter.

Spondylolysis

Repetitive bending forwards and backwards (flexing and extending) causes a stress on the area of the vertebra between the two joints, known as the pars interarticularis (part between two joints). This can result in the formation of a hairline crack, or stress fracture. This, of course, gives the player pain, which comes on gradually, getting worse with playing and training. A study in Norway found that soccer was only second to team handball in causing this injury. It most commonly involves the fifth lumbar vertebra.

The diagnosis is made by examination, and X-ray investigation. A plain X-ray of the lumbar spine, taken in the oblique position, may help, but an isotope bone scan will show the area as 'hot'. A bone scan involves the injection of a small amount of the radioactive element technetium, which delivers about the same radiation as a chest X-ray. The technetium is taken up by the cells that remodel bone when it is stressed. In a stress fracture, the bone is trying to heal itself, and becomes more active at this site. This is the cause of the 'hot spot'. To confirm the size of the damage, a CT scan is recommended.

In young people, this area of bone is the growing area. As mentioned in the section about bones in Chapter 3, this is more prone to damage by repetitive trauma, and these stresses may prevent the bone from fusing at puberty. There may be some back pain in adolescence, which is put down to 'growing pains'. However, later on in a soccer career the pain may return, and a spondylolysis found. These can be on one side, or both sides of the vertebra.

There is no first aid treatment as such. When the player presents with this injury, the relevant examination and investigation will define its extent. Treatment consists of rest until the pain settles, and a period of stability exercises to prevent excessive strain on the area when flexing and extending. If the player gets back to training and playing but the pain returns, there are various types of injection that may help return. Surgery is preserved for the few that have persistent pain and loss of function.

Spondylolisthesis

If the ring of the vertebra is not complete, as with a spondylolysis, the continuing pressure on the vertebra can force the front and back parts of the vertebra to move apart. This is a spondylolisthesis. This movement, or slip, is graded from grade 1 to 5. Grading aids accurate management and prognosis. The likely need of surgery to fix the crack in the vertebra is greater the higher the grade.

The cause of this problem is the failure, during puberty, of the arch of the vertebra to fuse. With a stress fracture, healing does not take place, and the bones slip apart.

Treatment is the same as with spondylolysis. Examination in this case may show a 'step' in the lumbar spine. This can be easily felt by running the fingers down the spine, with the player standing.

Core stability

This is a mode of rehabilitation that is important in spondylolisthesis, and in preventing recurrence.

As already mentioned, excessive movement of the spine can be one cause of injury, and it is therefore imperative with all types of back injury that this excess is restricted. With excessive flexion and extension, the vertebrae rock and rotate on the intervertebral discs. Sport probably causes more of this action than the human spine can generally withstand. It can affect the discs, the facet joints, and the vertebra itself. Similarly, excessive pelvic movement will have an action on the spine, and compound the excessive movement, and this time in different planes. Unless a way can be devised to halt this attrition, the sporting population will be left with ailing backs, and a trip to the doctor will be fruitless. This is where core stability comes in (*see* Chapter 12).

There are muscles around the abdomen and the pelvis that hold the lumbar spine still. These muscles exert less power if the player sustains a back injury of any kind, and the player enters a vicious cycle of excessive spinal and pelvic movement, attritional damage, and weaker reflex muscles. The way to reverse this cycle is to re-train the muscles to gain spinal and pelvic stability once more.

A group of special exercises can be undertaken to promote this stability. The muscles are reflex in their action, and as such, are more difficult to 'switch on'. To start this process, a qualified physiotherapist should be consulted. They may use ultrasound biofeedback and examination techniques to show the player how to use these muscles. This process will eventually result in the core muscles acting automatically to prevent excessive spinal movement, and hence attritional wear of the spinal structures.

Prolapsed Intervertebral Disc

During low jumping, the pressure at the third lumbar vertebra increases by 40% above the norm; for rotation, 20% greater. The force and intensity experienced in soccer can only make pressure on the lower spine worse.

Any action that puts excessive force on the disc can cause damage to the outer rim (annulus fibrosus), and allow the central viscous liquid (nucleus pulposus) to increase the pressure on the rim itself or even to ooze out through a small crack. The very strong ligaments around the spine limit the spread of this liquid. If there is pressure on the nerve where it exits from the vertebra, the player will feel pain in the distribution of that nerve root. As the lumbar spine is where the roots that form the sciatic nerve exit, this pain is called sciatica. There are differing severities of this condition, from mild to crippling.

Occasionally, a player has to be carried from the field with this injury. The incident causing the prolapse may be innocuous enough, but the player may be in agony. Although this is an unusual injury, a full examination should be carried out to determine whether there is any compromise of the nerve. If this is the case, a neurological opinion should be sought urgently. An MRI scan will confirm the extent of the injury, and appropriate action can be taken.

Treatment for this is most commonly 'at leisure', that is, the player will present after training or playing, with pain but not agonising pain. The same routine should be followed, and if necessary an MRI scan should

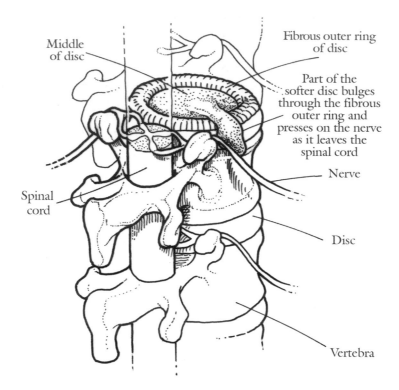

Lumbar spine prolapse.

be carried out to delineate the injury. With the help of the examination and scan, treatment can be aimed specifically at the site of injury. This will take the form of pain management with analgesia and NSAIDs, and the slow introduction of core stability exercises. Most of these injuries will take six to twelve weeks to make good, depending on the extent. If there is scant improvement in this time, and there is no other pathology, epidural or intra-foraminal injection of steroid can be undertaken. This often settles down the residual local inflammation, and allows the nerve to move more freely, and without this irritation the pain subsides. The player may need more than one injection before symptoms disappear completely.

Recurrence is always possible, but the maintenance of core stability exercises will reduce its likelihood.

The temptation is always to stop the exercises if the symptoms disappear. In professional soccer, these exercises are built into the training, so that no one can say they forgot them. It is more difficult for the recreational player with less time. One way to maintain them is to integrate them into other daily activities, waiting for the bus, at work, and so on.

Facet Joint Disruption

The facet joints are illustrated above. As stated before, these are situated just behind the opening which houses the spinal cord. The spinal cord itself stops at about the level of the first lumbar vertebra, but the nerves continue down to exit at the lower lumbar vertebra, and then to form the sciatic nerve. This collection of nerves is called the cauda equine (horse's tail).

The position of the facet joints means that if they become disrupted they can cause similar nerve pressure symptoms (sciatica) as intervertebral disc prolapse. The mechanism can also be very similar, causing a diagnostic dilemma. Rotation or bending backwards (extension), especially backwards and sideways at the same time, causes pressure on this joint. This joint has a structure very similar to the large joints in the body, but is much smaller. It has a capsule and the surfaces are covered in a smooth membrane (hyaline cartilage). The joint can swell, just like the knee joint does, when traumatized. The swelling presses on the nerve, causing sciatica. The irritation of the joint also causes pain that is perceived locally, that is, in the back.

Careful examination by an experienced physician or physiotherapist can usually diagnose this condition. However, the symptoms and signs of disc pathology, facet joint pathology, spondylolysis and spondylolisthesis can be very similar. Radiological investigation with X-ray, bone scan and MRI or CT scan can help to unpick the tangle.

Pain management is the cornerstone of treatment, with NSAIDs playing a big part. The joint should settle in two to four weeks, and core stability measures can be instituted. Occasionally, the joint remains painful, and in this case, an injection of steroid and anaesthetic, guided by CT scan, can be of benefit.

Core stability exercises will make sure that this has less of a chance of recurrence. The best results for core stability are gained when the player has minimal pain, so there is good incentive to intervene to eliminate symptoms.

CHAPTER 18

Injuries to the Hips, Pelvis and Groin

Injuries to the hip and groin area are common in soccer, amounting to 8% of all injuries, and cause many difficulties. The area is one of transition: the lower borders of the abdomen, and the upper borders of the leg meet and cross here. In soccer it is obviously an important zone.

Normal function of the hip joint is essential in soccer. The muscles used in locomotion use the pelvis or the lumbar spine as their anchor when moving. The muscle that lifts the hip during running and walking (flexing the hip), the ilio-psoas, runs from the lumbar spine, down through the pelvis to the top of the thighbone (femur). When it contracts, the thigh is lifted. Similarly, the various parts of the muscle responsible for kicking, the quadriceps, at the front of the thigh, originate at the front of the pelvis. The same can be said of the hamstring muscles that are situated at the back of the thigh and the adductor muscles that pull the leg towards the middle. This action is an essential part of sprinting. The fact that the pelvis or lumbar spine is the anchor of so many muscles causes problems in the muscles and their tendons, as well as the

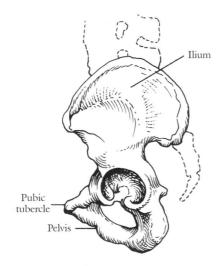

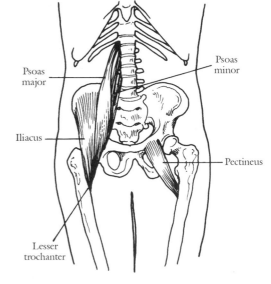

The hip joint.

162

sites of their attachments, both on the pelvis, and on the bones of the leg. If there is a lack of stability, excessive movement of the lumbar spine and pelvis can also cause injury.

The problem of muscular injury is compounded in some cases because some of the muscles cross two joints as they run their course, such as the rectus femoris muscle at the front of the thigh. The joints may not move in the same planes during movement, so this requires the muscle to function in a complex way, leaving it open to injury. Complicating things still further is the fact that pain in the groin and hip area may be radiated pain, caused by pressure on a nerve in the back, similar to sciatica, but the pain stays in the groin rather than radiating further down.

HIP JOINT INJURIES

The hip joint is a ball and socket joint, and one that is very stable: it has to be, as it supports the weight of the body. The 'ball' is the top, or head, of the femur (thighbone), and the socket is called the acetabulum. Just like the shoulder joint, its socket has a rim of fibrous cartilage-like tissue around it. This is called the labrum acetabulare (in the shoulder it is the labrum glenoidale).

It is important to think of all ages when talking about hip injuries. Soccer is a sport played by children as well as adults, and by both sexes. Some hip injuries are age specific.

Perthes Disease

Called Legg-Calve-Perthes disease in full, this is an unusual condition, but an important one to recognize. It is a disease of the hip that affects mostly four- to seven-year-olds, more boys than girls. Usually the children are small and underdeveloped. The cause is unknown, but what happens is that the blood vessels supplying the head of the femur shut down. This causes 'avascular necrosis', which means that the bone dies (necroses) because of loss of blood supply.

As one would expect, there are differing severities of this, and outcome depends on severity. With the mildest form, the head of the femur can recover completely. With the worst of this disease, the player may end up with a hip replacement, but if there is early recognition and appropriate treatment, this may be delayed until the fifth decade of life. Of course, if a player presents with this disease, it may be that their playing career may be shortened, or even prematurely ended.

Hip disease in children can present commonly as knee pain, and confuse the examiner. Remember that in children the complaint may be of knee pain, but examination of the knee may be normal.

There is a lack of hip rotational movement, with pain. There may be shortening of the limb, and a loss of muscle due to disuse. X-ray examination will show a characteristic distortion of the normal architecture of the hip joint.

Treatment is under the auspices of orthopaedic surgeons, who may follow these players for many years, planning care with the player as time passes.

As far as prevention, and prevention of recurrence is concerned, the lack of real knowledge of cause means that prevention is impossible. Epidemiologically, there are some common factors, but these do not come into the scope of this book, being public health issues.

Slipped Upper Femoral Epiphysis (SUFE)

As described in Chapter 3, bones grow by putting down new bone, layer upon layer, thereby making the bone longer. The laying down process occurs at the growth plate, which usually sits between the end and shaft of the bone. In the case of SUFE, the top of the femur slips off the growth plate. The movement is small, but this causes a change in the mechanics of the joint. It is more common in boys, and occurs at 11–13 years of age in girls, 12–14 in boys.

The player may present with knee pain. The hip should always be examined in cases of knee pain. There is a loss of internal rotation with pain when forcing this movement. Ultrasound examination can show an effusion in the joint, and in skilled hands demonstrate the slip. X-ray examination will also show the slip, as will an MRI scan.

The treatment is surgical, with replacement of the hip. The other unaffected side may be done at the same time, as there is a risk the same will happen. It may take up to two years for the player to return to play. It is, again, associated with premature onset of degenerative disease of the joint, although this is unpredictable.

As far as prevention, and prevention of recurrence is concerned, there are some associations of this disease with constitutional factors. It is also associated with some medical syndromes, but is impossible to predict and, therefore, unpreventable. After fixation there is no recurrence.

Torn Labrum Acetabulare

This structure may be torn during exercise, when the joint is forced in a way that is outside its normal range of movement. The rim of cartilage gets caught in the joint as it moves, and tears. This torn cartilage then gets in the way of normal hip movements.

Often, the player feels 'something go'. After the original pain settles, there may be a 'catch' or pain when the hip gets into a certain position. Examination can mimic the hip position that brings the pain on, but rotation of the hip inwards, especially when the leg is pointing away from the body, usually brings on pain. This can be a difficult injury to diagnose. Plain X-rays are normal. MRI with dye injected into the joint is the most accurate diagnostic tool.

First aid treatment is directed at pain relief. The nature of this injury is that it is often difficult to diagnose immediately after suffering it. After a few days, it becomes more obvious what the injury is, and the correct investigations can be arranged. If the diagnosis is confirmed, surgery is the only option. The cartilage is trimmed, and normal function returns after surgery.

As a traumatic injury, this is largely unpreventable. However, if the muscles around the hip are trained to stabilize the movements around the hip, they may have a protective function. This is theoretical though, and is not backed up by evidence.

Bursitis

The structure and function of bursas (bursae) is dealt with in Chapter 3. There are multiple bursae around the hip, and all can get injured and cause pain.

Trochanteric bursitis

The bony prominence called the greater trochanter is located at the outside of the thigh, and there is a bursa acting as protection for the muscle–tendon structure that runs across it.

The bursa may become injured if it is irritated by the repeated movement of the muscle–tendon, or by local trauma. The way that the muscle–tendon irritates the bursa may be related to biomechanical issues, or by unusually tight muscles, or both.

A player with this condition complains of tenderness over the greater trochanter. If this area is prodded, the player's pain will be reproduced. An ultrasound scan may show the enlarged bursa. Of course, the examination process should include a biomechanical assessment, sometimes using video analysis of the way the player runs. This may help in the overall management and prevention of this injury.

If the biomechanical evaluation shows that their way of running predisposes the player to this injury, a podiatrist may prescribe orthoses for the shoes that change the way the foot acts during running. If there are tight muscles contributing to this injury, the player will be given a stretch routine. As long as the physiotherapist and physician are happy that these things have been addressed, steroid injection, guided by ultrasound scan into the appropriate area, is the treatment of choice.

If implicated, attention to the biomechanics relating to running will help prevent recurrence. Protection with a 'doughnut' of felt or sponge may help attenuate the amount of trauma sustained. Goalkeepers often need this type of protection, until they are allowed to rest after the season. Often, there is no obvious reason for this injury, and without this it is difficult to prevent.

Ilio-psoas bursitis

The main hip flexor (the muscle that lifts the thigh up when going up the stairs), is called the ilio-psoas. It effects hip flexion via its attachment on the lesser trochanter near the top of the femur, or thighbone. As the tendon meets the bone, there is a bursa to protect the tendon from attritional wear as it butts up against the bone.

Similarly to greater trochanteric bursitis, this kind of bursitis is caused by tight muscle groups causing trapping of the bursa, thereby inflaming it, and local trauma. If there is local trauma, the case history alone may lead to diagnosis, but the onset is often insidious.

This is a deep structure, and there are many others around this area. This means that diagnosis can be less than straightforward. Examination is largely aimed at excluding other causes of hip and groin pain. If the hip joint is flexed to 90° and the knee taken across the body, this may squash the bursa and reproduce the symptoms. Testing the flexibility of the psoas muscle itself may demonstrate a tight muscle which, when under tension, may cause pain by squashing the bursa.

Imaging with X-rays is unhelpful, but ultrasound scans and MRI scans may help. The diagnosis often remains a clinical one, that is one made by taking a thorough case history and undertaking a thorough examination.

Treatment comprises resting the player and making sure that the ilio-psoas muscle is flexible, which may take the pressure off the bursa. If this does not work, the bursa can be injected with a steroid under direct ultrasound guidance. More than one may be needed.

Keeping the hip flexor muscles stretched may help prevent recurrence. When embarking upon such a course, the complete pelvic–spinal stability must be addressed. It may be that the hip flexor muscle has become tight because the local stability required it. By addressing the lumbar spine and pelvic control in a global sense, the muscle concerned may stay stretched and flexible, rather than re-attain its previous length, and go on to cause ilio-psoas bursitis again.

Complaints of lower-back pain are most often the result of muscle strains or ligament sprains and usually respond well to conservative management. However, persistent or recurrent back pain or nerve root symptoms should warrant a further diagnostic evaluation. Groin injuries are perhaps the most common of injuries to the lower trunk, pelvis, and/or upper leg in soccer. Chronic groin pain is often encountered in soccer players and is likely caused by the biomechanics of forceful kicking in which abdominal muscles and hip flexors and adductors are repetitively stressed.

The Sacro-iliac Joint (SIJ)

The SIJ is located, as the name would suggest, where the sacrum, and ilium of the pelvis, meet. It has long been the subject of debate, centred around whether, and how much, it moves. Most clinicians these days accept that it moves, and can cause symptoms, but this movement in no way mirrors that experienced in other joints. The limit of rotation in this joint has been measured at 5–8mm, in those patients without back pain. Sacro-iliac pain has been reported to radiate anywhere around the upper thigh and groin, and will continue to confuse everyone concerned. As age increases, the joint becomes stiffer; hence movement will, similarly, be less. Its position, being the 'keystone' in connecting the spine to the pelvis, means that any uneven or excessive forces are likely to cause injury.

Not only is the SIJ prone to injury, it can also be a target in inflammatory conditions. Although being a rheumatological condition rather than a sporting injury it is outside the scope of this book, it is mentioned here because its symptoms can be overlooked by being attributed to the rough and tumble of soccer, and the age of onset is similar to that of the normal sporting population.

Sacro-iliitis

Trauma may cause disruption of the joint, as with any joint. This trauma may be direct, or be made by using the thigh as a lever. If the hip is abducted, and direct trauma applied to the knee, the transmitted forces may cause impaction and rotation of the SIJ, causing pain.

SIJ pain is also produced by the repetitive, less forceful, trauma that can be attributed to biomechanical and postural features inherent

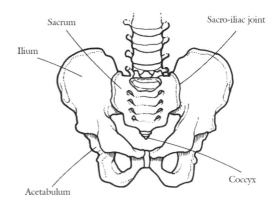

The sacro-iliac joint.

to the athlete. For instance, one leg being longer than the other may put an uneven force across the SIJ, and cause pain during or after exercise.

The SIJ is often a focus for inflammation from conditions such as ankylosing spondylitis and psoriatic arthritis. These conditions have a hereditary factor, and probably environmental factors. The onset of these diseases is usually in adolescence, and often in those who are active. The feature is usually that the pain is worse with rest rather than exercise. Pain often wakes the sufferer early in the morning, but by the time they have left the house, the pain is easing. There may be the presence of a genetic marker that can be measured in a blood sample, but it is not always present even in those who have the illness. It is called HLAB27, and is one of a number of 'HLA antigens' that aid diagnosis in a range of conditions.

We have briefly discussed that the SIJ can cause diagnostic problems, because of the overlapping of symptoms. A full examination by the team physician or physiotherapist will usually be able to tease out the diagnosis.

A plain X-ray may be helpful, and if there is diagnostic doubt about whether the SIJ is implicated in the production of the player's symptoms, then injection under X-ray guidance of dye and anaesthetic may be of help. If this is done, and the player's pain is reduced, the SIJ can rightly be accused.

An MRI scan will show inflammation in the peri-articular tissues, which may be absent on plain X-ray. Isotope bone scanning will show increased uptake of the radioactive dye in the SIJ. Both these imply that the SIJ is inflamed, and that there is a strong likelihood that this is the seat of a player's symptoms.

For traumatic problems, early mobilization under the protection of NSAIDs will benefit. Physiotherapy with mobilization of the affected joint will aid recovery. Inflammatory problems are dealt with using NSAIDs, and exercise. Without the exercise, the ligaments within the joint become stiffer and more painful. Exercise keeps these ligaments loose, less stiff, and therefore less painful. The anti-inflammatories may be enough to dampen the inflammation, but the player should be under the care of a rheumatologist, and regularly reviewed.

As far as prevention is concerned, biomechanical assessment prior to exercise participation may be effective in preventing the onset of these symptoms. However, there are pitfalls, as mentioned previously. Changing the biomechanical make-up of a player without reported symptoms that may be attributable to any biomechanical issue, can cause its own problems, hence clouding the diagnostic process.

Certainly, secondary prevention of SIJ dysfunction should include careful assessment of the biomechanics of the player concerned. Leg length differences can lead to SIJ pain, but this is not a universal finding, hence difficult to predict.

Piriformis syndrome

The piriformis muscle arises from the front of the sacrum, and runs outwards, through the sciatic, notch before inserting into the top of the greater trochanter of the femur (thighbone). This is the bony prominence felt high up on the outside of the thigh. The sciatic nerve also comes out of the sciatic notch, and does so underneath the piriformis muscle. This means that if the muscle is tight or swollen for any reason, for instance after trauma, the sciatic nerve is pressed upon, causing pain. These symptoms can easily mimic the sciatica that has its origin in the lumbar spine from, for example, a bulging intervertebral disc. The sciatic nerve irritation symptoms are often accompanied by local pain in the buttock area, although not always.

Local trauma to the buttock may cause bleeding and swelling within the muscle belly. This in turn causes compression of the underlying nerve. If the muscle is naturally tight, which can happen if the muscle is highly trained and conditioned, similar pressure may be applied to the nerve, causing pain and a tingling sensation in the distribution of the sciatic nerve. Occasionally, the sciatic nerve runs a slightly different course, and this makes pressure upon it more likely.

Diagnosis can be very difficult, especially if the symptoms are solely of sciatica. The history may be one of local buttock trauma, with no other precipitating factors. If this is so, piriformis syndrome should be considered. However, because of the nature of contact sport, it can be hard for the player to remember every bump and knock they sustain.

Examination may demonstrate sciatic nerve irritation, with the slump test and the straight leg raise test bringing on the symptoms. In this case, the first culprit to suspect is the lumbar spine area. If investigations are fruitless, other causes must be sought for sciatic nerve pressure. The acronym FAIR has been used to describe the mode of examining for piriformis syndrome: F (hip Flexion), A (Adduction), and IR (Internal Rotation). The way to achieve this is to lie the patient on his side, with the affected side upwards. The affected side hip should be flexed, and the knee allowed to fall, with gravity, onto the couch, or over the edge of the couch, so achieving the FAIR posture. The examiner then examines the buttock, just behind the hip joint. Pressure at this area exacerbates the symptoms, and the diagnosis is made. Electromyography may be undertaken to demonstrate sciatic nerve dysfunction. Radiology, unless there is a high suspicion, is largely unhelpful.

The initial treatment is physiotherapy, with massage, and a stretching programme. At this time, a core stability programme should be instigated to ensure permanent alleviation of symptoms. Occasionally surgical intervention may be required, although injection of botulinum toxin and/or steroids and local anaesthetic may be tried.

If the underlying cause is trauma, prevention is of course impossible. Muscle tightness can be treated by a stretching and massage programme, which should be part of normal conditioning. Of course, if the sciatic nerve is sited such that it becomes more easily susceptible to pressure, there is no preventive strategy that will be effective, except to say that a stretching and conditioning programme becomes even more important. Bear in mind that there is no way of knowing whether a player's anatomy is of this kind.

Clicking or Snapping Hip

There are two main causes of this problem, which can be painful and distressing to the player. The first is due to the psoas muscle. This muscle (with iliacus) is the main flexor of the hip, and is used in ambulation of all types. It comes from the side of the lumbar spine and travels down through the pelvis, and into the femur (thighbone), just inside the hip joint itself. In this complaint, the tendon of the muscle can slip across the edge of the bone near where it inserts into the top of the femur and causes a snap. It usually happens at about 45° of hip flexion. This can be due to a tight muscle, or due to the swelling of the bursa that sits by the muscle insertion to protect it.

The other common cause is the ilio-tibial band flicking across the greater trochanter on the outside of the upper thigh. The ilio-tibial band, or ITB, arises at the iliac crest, and runs down the outside of the thigh, and inserts into the outside of the tibia or shinbone.

Tightness in the ITB may be due to bio-mechanical issues, often associated with high-arched feet. Sports associated with repetitive movement patterns also predispose to this condition. Hence, runners tend to suffer this condition more than footballers.

Diagnosis is made from the case history. If the psoas is the cause, the clicking or snapping is experienced 'deep' in the groin, and at the front of the groin area. During examination, it becomes evident that the muscle on that side is tighter than on the other. When comparing muscle flexibility, stretching the muscle can reproduce the symptoms. If the ITP is the problem, the clicking or snapping is experienced on the outside of the thigh, and can be reproduced when stretching the ITB over the greater trochanter. Pressing over this reproduces discomfort or pain, which worsens as the game or training session progresses.

Treatment is rest, and a stretching programme which will usually effect cure. It is vital that the issue of core stability should be addressed. Often these muscle groups become tight because of poor central stability. The player should be fully assessed by a podiatrist to examine the role of biomechanics in this.

Soccer players spend their playing and training life in partial flexion. That is to say that they are bent forwards, in a state of readi-ness, often on their toes. In this situation, the hip flexors and ITBs will become tighter and are prone to causing snapping or clicking. A programme of stretching and conditioning is the only way to prevent this.

Psoas Bursitis

As explained earlier, a bursa (pl.= bursae) is a sac of fluid that is found between a tendon and a bone, in the place where the tendon inserts into the bone. The psoas muscle is the main flexor of the hip joint, so it inserts into the top of the femur, just to the inside, and below the joint itself. As the muscle inserts into the bone, it is protected by the psoas bursa. This bursa can become inflamed, and swell. As there is no space to enlarge into, the swelling causes pressure on the tendon, giving pain.

Tightness in the psoas muscle can cause friction to the bursa, setting up a 'vicious circle' of inflammation and increasing swelling in the bursa. It was mentioned that soccer players spend most time in a 'flexed' position (bent forward, with hips and knees bent), and it is easy to imagine that the hip flexor (psoas) muscle may become tight. Local trauma to the front of the groin can cause swelling to the bursa, and once again, the vicious circle begins.

This can be difficult, as there is a multitude of structures in this area. When examining anything in the groin, it is important to remember that pressure on the nerve roots of the lumbar spine can be related to groin pain. The groin area receives its nerve supply from the first lumbar (L1) root. Careful examination of the lumbar spine often reveals an origin for the player's complaint.

If the problem is true psoas bursitis, causing

pressure upon it reproduces the player's symptoms. With the player lying on the back, flex the hip and knee to 90° then bring the knee across the body. This compresses the bursa, and reproduces the pain. Local tenderness can also be felt, but can be difficult to interpret. Scanning the area, either with ultrasound or MRI, can sometimes demonstrate fluid at the site of the bursa, but not always, and a negative scan does not negate the diagnosis.

As implied above, a course of stretching and stability will reduce pressure on the bursa, allowing it to settle. During the period of treatment, NSAIDs will help to reduce swelling. If this does not work, the bursa can be injected with steroid and local anaesthetic. This should ideally be done using ultrasound or CT guidance, ensuring the best outcome.

Because of the inherent posture necessary for performance in soccer, working on the tight muscle groups is the only way to aid prevention. Players need to be persuaded into an ongoing stretching and stability programme.

Inflammatory Arthropathy of the Hip

Any joint can become inflamed. If this is secondary to trauma, the cause is self-evident. However, occasionally the immune system can cause inflammation by attacking native tissues. This is called auto-immune inflammation. The hip joint, like the sacro-iliac joint (see above) can become inflamed in this way.

The lack of trauma may point to the diagnosis. If the team physician or physiotherapist feels that the case history, symptoms and examination findings do not add up to a 'normal' hip picture, blood tests and X-rays or other scans should be arranged. Prompt referral to a rheumatologist is mandatory.

Gilmore's Groin or Conjoint Tendon Disruption

There has been much debate over the origin of this condition. There are many ways to explain it, but to explain the anatomy may help to understand where the problem is, and the reason for the type of symptoms experienced by players.

There is a small opening (the superficial inguinal ring) in the lower abdomen where, in males, the testicle exits the abdominal cavity, and descends into the forming scrotum. The opening is there in females also, but smaller, due to the differing pelvic shapes between the sexes. (Hence, this condition is more common in males.)

Surrounding this opening is a structure called the conjoint tendon. It is not a tendon like the tendons that attach muscle to bone, but more of a thickening of the covering of the muscles in the front of the abdomen.

This injury is not exclusive to footballers. It is more common in those players who pivot more, perhaps playing a centre field position. There is a feeling that those with better core (central) stability have less chance of suffering this condition. However, there have been no wide-ranging prospective studies to test this. Invariably, if the player complains of this, and the state of their stability is measured, it is difficult to know which came first, the condition or the lack of stability.

Diagnosis is made by the examiner, and can be uncomfortable for the patient. Examination of the superficial inguinal ring reproduces the player's pain. Scans and X-rays may show inflammation in the area, but are often unhelpful. Herniography, where there is a radio-opaque dye injected into the abdominal cavity, can be helpful. In this procedure, dye can leak outside the abdominal cavity through the superficial inguinal ring. This leakage is then picked up on plain X-ray. The diagnosis is often delayed, and players can be suffering for some time.

In keeping with a relatively newly identified condition, there has also been debate about the treatment. Some advocate a course of core stability exercises, in the hope that controlling excessive movement may stop disruption of the conjoint tendon. Surgery, if the diagnosis is correct, is curative, and the player can be back on the pitch in six weeks.

As intimated above, there is a feeling that better control of abdominal and pelvic musculature may prevent the excessive movements experienced by these tissues whilst playing. This is certainly the only strategy for prevention of this condition at present.

The thigh is the powerhouse in able-bodied sport, with the largest muscle groups in the body, the quadriceps (at the front), and the hamstrings (at the back). With this knowledge, it is no surprise that these muscles get injured regularly. There are intrinsic injuries, such as in a pull or strain when the muscle is over-reached in some way, and extrinsic ones, such as the trauma of receiving a kick.

THE GROIN

The groin is an area of transition of body zones, and as such is prone to injury. The groin is the border between:

• the abdomen and the thigh
• the pelvis and lumbar spine
• the hip joint and femur.

Crossing this border are the various components necessary for ambulation. First there are the muscles, anchored to the lower lumbar spine and pelvis, and inserted into the particular bones that need to be moved to allow motion. The nerves to supply these muscles come from the lower lumbar and sacral areas, and, with the associated blood vessels, also run through the groin area.

Within a very small cross-sectional area, therefore, there are many structures that can be injured during soccer, whether by trauma, strains, sprains, tears or fractures. The diagnosis of the cause of pain and dysfunction in this region can be difficult, as more than one problem may be present at any one time. Trying to pinpoint pain with touch alone means that more than one structure is pushed upon, confusing the diagnosis.

Many players will complain of 'groin pain', and the medical team must make sure that they consider all local anatomical structures, but not forget more distant structures (for example, nerves from the lumbar spine), as possible culprits.

Adductor Muscle Injury

The word adduct has the opposite meaning to abduct. To abduct is to take away (like kidnapping), so to adduct is to bring back. The adductor muscles bring the thigh, and hence the leg, back towards the middle of the body. If one tries to press one's knees together, this is achieved by using the group of muscles called the adductor muscles.

These muscles are used in kicking, but also in sprinting. A jogger makes two lines of prints, one for each foot, whereas a sprinter makes one line of prints (check it out on a beach). The faster we run, the closer to a single line our footprints get. This is due to the action of the adductor muscles. These muscles have their origin, or anchor, at the pubic bone, which is at the lowest part of the abdomen, in the middle. They attach at various points on the femur, the lowest point being just above the line of the knee joint.

It follows that, as sprinting and kicking are integral to soccer, the adductor muscles ought to be prone to injury, and they are. All soccer teams experience this type of injury with relentless regularity. This may change, as research has been done on how to avoid this troublesome injury.

Kicking is the major cause of the injury. The act of kicking – forcing a ball in a certain direction, using a foot – involves many muscle groups and individual muscles. Some styles of kicking, like those involved in trying to bend the ball, may use different muscles more than other styles. If the kick is more forceful than usual, or the player is not properly 'set' for the kick, muscles are then required to act at a mechanical disadvantage, and hence may be susceptible to injury. This is the case with the adductor muscles when kicking. One of the adductor muscles is injured more often in kicking than the others. This is the adductor longus, although the other adductor muscles can be involved. Reaching or lunging for a ball as it goes past during play can cause an overstretching of the adductors, causing tearing.

As the game goes on, fatigue may become a factor in this type of injury. There is no test yet that determines the amount of fatigue players, or their muscles, are experiencing, but certainly adductor injuries often happen late in the game, in the act of kicking. Occasionally, an adductor muscle can be pulled off its attachment at the symphysis pubis. This is more common in adolescent players, but is not unknown in those players with more mature skeletons.

The diagnosis is made when the player feels 'something go' on the inside of the thigh, and this alerts the medical team. Although this is the usual scenario, on occasion the player will feel the groin become tight during the game or training session.

Examination must involve all the elements that can cause pain in this area of the body. The adductors will have a reduced range of motion, be painful when stretched, and upon contraction when resisted. There will be a painful region when the muscles are probed. This is often where the muscle–tendon is attached in the upper groin, but may be at the site of transition of the muscle and tendon, 3–5cm from the attachment of the muscle. X-rays may show an avulsion fracture if this is present, although this is unusual.

Since the advent of MRI scanning, accurate diagnosis, and hence prognosis and treatment, have improved greatly. The muscle will show inflammatory fluid or haemorrhage in the region of the injury, and the rest of the anatomical region can be assessed to ascertain whether the injury has affected any other part of the area. Remember, the region of the groin, including the adductors, can be difficult to assess, and it can save a lot of heartache if it is realized early on that there is more than one pathology present.

Although MRI is very useful in a global assessment, ultrasound scanning can outline, and more accurately grade, muscle disruption. It can be useful used in tandem with MRI, and can offer the most accurate prognosis, with clinical assessment, that can be made.

When considering prevention, remember that lack of strength, with respect to muscle balance and imbalance, and lack of stretch are the most important reasons for sustaining adductor strains. At the signing, or pre-season assessment, the adductor muscle group should be carefully considered, and range of movement and strength be measured. There is no 'normal' range of motion, but it seems obvious that in a sport where large ranges of motion are needed to play effectively, a lack of range may lead to injury and perhaps ineffectiveness. The latter may curtail a promising career as much as an injury might. The question of strength is a difficult one. The adductors are part of the integrated muscular system around the lower pelvis. Strengthening them alone may leave other muscles and soft tissues at risk due to the over-activity of the adductor group.

Osteitis Pubis

The pubic symphysis consists of the two pubic bones that meet centrally. It can be felt at the lowest part of the abdomen, just above the genital area. The joint between the two pubic bones has a pad of fibrocartilage (like that found in the knee and the shoulder), and is bound together by strong ligaments. It moves and is the only part of the ring of the pelvis that does so to any degree. The sacro-iliac joint does move, but minimally, and only in one direction.

The groin area is complicated and it can be difficult to isolate the site of pain and injury. In the recent past, many have begun to see groin pain and injury as part of a spectrum of injury of the area that could be described generically as 'groin injury'. This is similar to other generic terms such as 'exercise-induced lower limb pain', which now includes even stress fractures. This allows clinicians to understand the whole area, and look at it holistically when looking for cause and cure.

In professional football, nearly all players will have some degenerative changes associated with the pubic symphysis. Not all players will have symptoms, however, and degeneration of the joint found on X-ray should not necessarily be taken as needing treatment.

This joint becomes inflamed and degenerated in footballers because of longstanding irritation from playing, and training, nearly every day for perhaps twenty years. The act of kicking compresses and rotates the joint, causing cumulative shearing and wearing.

In the groin area all the structures are functionally, as well as anatomically, related. The consequence of this is that if there are any asymmetries or lack of mobility or strength, this may focus on the symphysis pubis. Lack of hip rotation, either from developmental causes, tight muscle groups, or degenerative change, may cause excessive movement across the symphysis pubis, leading to attritional wear of the joint. Excessive muscle action of the adductor muscles can cause similar wear by excessive traction on their attachment to the pubic bones.

The fact that the ring of the pelvis is normally stable means that excessive shearing forces will be caused if the sacro-iliac joint is unstable. This is unusual, but after trauma, such as a road traffic accident, there may be such a disruption of the intra-articular ligaments of the SIJ, resulting in instability.

The nerves supplying this joint arise in the lumbar spine, and if there is any irritation of these nerves, such as from disc or facet joint pathology, the player may feel pain around the pubic symphysis. Athletes from all sports, including soccer, may have one leg longer than the other. This can obviously cause shearing at the symphysis pubis during running. Inflammatory arthritis has been described above in association with the sacro-iliac joint. This can also occur in the pubic symphysis.

Infection has been described in the pubic symphysis, usually associated with surgical procedures, gynaecological in women, and prostate problems in men. Obviously, if the patient has recently had surgery, this has to be suspected. However, there are a couple of reports in the literature of infection with no obvious cause, so although this is rare, it must be considered.

In making a diagnosis, the case history of the pain and its onset is important. The pain usually comes on gradually, gets worse with exercise, and can take a day or two to settle. The condition of the playing surface may have a bearing on the severity of the pain, with both hard and muddy or sticky playing fields making the pain worse.

The medical team will examine the mechanics of the player, including accurate leg length, as well as a close examination of the pelvic and groin area, before coming to a diagnosis of osteitis pubis. The diagnosis must be supported by positive radiological changes at the symphysis pubis.

Traditionally, since first described in the 1960s, the diagnosis has been made by plain X-ray, and isotope bone scanning. The X-ray changes are graded as:

STAGE 0 X-ray normal, but player has pain
STAGE 1 X-ray exam with typical 'moth-eaten' appearance in joint
STAGE 2 X-ray exam with deeper and asymmetric erosions
STAGE 3 X-ray showing an even more deformed symphysis with an established osteoarthritis and worsening moth-eaten appearance

STAGE 4 X-ray exam showing widespread degeneration of the joint, with bone overgrowth. There is severe irregularity of the joint.

'Flamingo' X-ray views, taken with the player standing on one foot, then the other, may show instability at the pubic symphysis, demonstrated by more than 2mm between one half of the joint and the other.

Paradoxically, all these grades may be accompanied by disabling symptoms or with minimal symptoms. It is easier to correlate symptoms with appearances of an isotope bone scan. This will show a hot spot over the area of the symphysis pubis, helping to confirm the diagnosis.

The advent of MRI has given more of an insight into the pathology of osteitis pubis. It allows the clinician to assess the bone, either side of the joint, as well as the adductor muscle insertions and the other pelvic structures. If there is any doubt, the lumbar spine may be scanned at the same time. MRI scanning of the pubic symphysis will show bone bruising, and any inflammation in the muscles or tendons. This confirms the diagnosis, and also allows for specific treatments.

Treatment will depend on the diagnosis. If there is an adductor problem that is revealed by examination and MRI scanning, treatment should be directed at this. If there is bone bruising associated with the pubic symphysis, the treatment traditionally has been rest, for up to three months. Recently however, pamidronate, which is a drug that modifies the way bone responds to inflammation, can be given. If given as a one-off intravenous dose, the recovery can be shortened to four weeks, rather than twelve weeks. Local injection of steroid may alleviate pain in a good proportion of patients with this injury, but administration can be painful.

Of course, any biomechanical issues must be addressed and dealt with, or treatment will be fruitless, as the irritation causing the problem will cause a recurrence. It is often the case that after treating the osteitis pubis, the central pain disappears, only to unveil a second problem, sometimes a groin or adductor disruption. Despite the impression that initial treatment will have cured the problem, the clinician should still be open to there being another local pathology. Of course, if there is a rheumatological or infective cause, these should be treated appropriately.

Assessing biomechanics as a primary preventative measure has many pitfalls. However, if the medical team are aware of the possible pathologies that may arise from biomechanical issues, intervention may be instigated at the first sign of a problem.

A stretching programme should ensure a good range of motion for the adductor muscles. The strength of the adductor muscles is also important. Pelvic muscle balance and stability is a must as a primary and a secondary prevention strategy. If the ground conditions are thought to be a pre-disposing factor, for instance hard grounds at certain times of the season, changing training routines will reduce the incidence.

CHAPTER 19

Injuries to the Thigh

The thigh is the powerhouse in able-bodied sport, with the largest muscle groups in the body, the quadriceps (at the front), and the hamstrings (at the back). With this knowledge, it is no surprise that these muscles get injured regularly. There are intrinsic injuries, such as in a pull or strain when the muscle is over-reached in some way, and extrinsic ones, such as the trauma of receiving a kick.

TORN QUADRICEPS

The quadriceps, compromising four large muscles in the front of the thigh, is the largest muscle group in the body. It sits at the front of the thigh, and is the antagonist to the hamstring muscle group. Hence, the quadriceps is the main extensor, or straightener of the knee. It does this via the large tendon that inserts into the upper front part of the shinbone. This tendon is protected by a large bone called a sesamoid. There are several sesamoid bones in the body, and they are present to protect large tendons from attritional wear. In this case, the sesamoid is called the knee-cap, or patella.

Rectus Femoris Strain

Although it is possible to pull any part of the muscle, the rectus femoris (known to

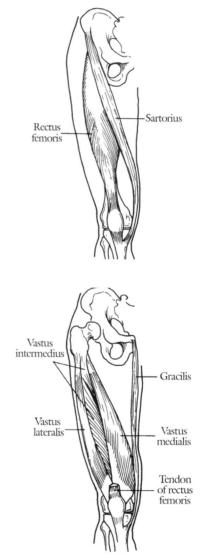

The quadriceps.

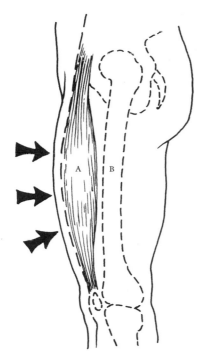

Common sites of quadriceps pulls.

The diagnosis is made from the case history and examination. An ultrasound or MRI scan will help to grade the extent of the tear or disruption, and hence lend more accuracy to prognosis.

In the first 48 hours, the muscle is treated by protecting it, preventing continuing stretching of the muscle. This may mean keeping the limb still, and non-weight bearing with the use of crutches. The area of the injury should be iced, compressed, and the leg elevated as much as is possible. If the continual stretching of the already disrupted muscle tear can be avoided, further injury can be prevented.

After 48 hours, active contraction, both concentric then eccentric, can be applied to the muscle, thereby ensuring that any scar tissue will be formed in the 'lines of force' of the muscle tendon unit. This is essential, as any scar tissue that forms skewed will have less tensile strength, and be susceptible to re-tearing. Rehabilitation will include looking at the biomechanics of the player's kicking action, and deciding whether there are ways in which muscle groups, especially those around the pelvis, contributed to the muscle tear.

Once any biomechanical issue is identified this must be addressed, and corrected if at all possible. It may be that there are reasons why it cannot be, for example in disabled players with neurological conditions.

Prevention will centre around adequate warm-up and length of the muscle concerned. A stretching programme is of paramount importance. Players need to know that they must never go out to warm-up and have a shot at goal as their first action.

some as the kicking muscle) is by far the most commonly affected. This muscle has its origin at two small sites just above the hip joint. It then runs down the front of the thigh, in the middle.

The rectus femoris is at risk of tearing because it runs across two joints, the hip and the knee, and more often tears at the site overlying the joint itself. In the action of kicking, the muscle is stretched when the leg is pulled back before kicking, the so-called back-lift. The thigh then moves forward as the foot accelerates towards the ball, but then stops whilst the foot 'catches up' just before striking the ball. At this stage, the muscle is at risk of tearing, and does so at the point overlying the hip joint. The player will feel 'something go' in the front of the thigh, with pain.

OTHER THIGH PROBLEMS

Meralgia Parasthetica

The skin on the front outside part of the front of the thigh has its nerve supply from a nerve that runs underneath the inguinal ligament and sometimes through one of the muscles in the thigh called the sartorius. On its course, it can become trapped and cause numbness or pain on the outside front of the thigh.

Local trauma to the area over the nerve can cause bruising around the nerve and stop it from working normally. The player will experience pain and tingling along the course of the nerve. Local pressure from tight shorts or underpants, or onset after surgery, perhaps for groin disruption, are other causes. Diabetes mellitus causes nerve damage, and rarely may present as meralgia parasthetica.

The case history, if taken carefully, will point to this diagnosis. However, confirmation will require nerve conduction studies. This will show that the nerve is not working properly, and where the pressure is. If there is not easy access to this investigation, local anaesthetic injection around the nerve as it appears from under the inguinal ligament will ablate the symptoms, hence confirming the suspicion. Urine should always be tested for glucose to exclude diabetes mellitus.

It is reasonable to try a local steroid injection in the first instance, as if there is some swelling, for whatever reason, it may respond to the anti-inflammatory action of this drug. If this is ineffective, then surgical decompression is required, but only if the symptoms are so troublesome as to interfere with playing and training. Of course, if the root cause is diabetes mellitus, this must be addressed, and one would expect the symptoms to disappear with time.

Myositis Ossificans

Myo = muscle, *itis* = inflammation, so myositis means inflammation of muscle. To ossify is to turn to bone, so myositis ossificans means inflammation of muscle that involves new bone formation. What happens in this condition is that, after trauma, there is bleeding into the muscle and disruption of some cells that surround the bone, and a process is set up with new bone being formed in the muscle itself. This is a temporary situation, but can be a real problem, as it can take some months to resolve.

The cause is mostly direct trauma. The classic injury is the 'dead leg', or 'crazy horse'. This is when a player's thigh is hit from the side, often by an opponent's knee. There are many reports in research literature describing myositis ossificans at various sites, not necessarily associated with sport, but with surgery, or repetitive movement. Muscle tears can also result in myositis ossificans, but less frequently so. After some time, the area becomes increasingly hard, and movement restricted.

It should be remembered that there are diseases such as tuberculosis and some tropical diseases that can cause bone formation in unexpected areas.

An X-ray or ultrasound scan will aid diagnosis, and although MRI is traditionally less helpful, more work is being done with MRI in the diagnosis and management of this condition, and it is being used more frequently.

Treatment has traditionally centred around rest, waiting, and surgery if there is no resolution. However, there is now more use of bisphosphonate drugs (such as pamidronate) to encourage resolution of the newly formed bone. This can still take time, and in élite players this wait can be unacceptable, so surgery is sometimes a preferred option. However, surgery can exacerbate rather than cure the problem.

Prevention, therefore, has to be the aim. The use of indomethacin early in cases of muscle trauma is known to reduce the incidence or amount of bone formation in myositis ossificans. In the case of a dead leg or crazy horse, if the player cannot bend the knee to 90°, they should be given indomethacin by prescription, and all massage avoided for at least 48 hours. Having a high index of suspicion will lead the medical team to investigate and instigate treatment early.

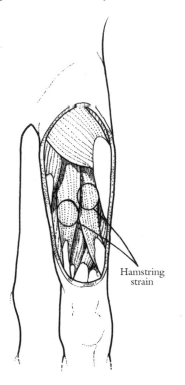

Hamstring strain

Common sites of hamstring pulls.

Hamstring Injury

The hamstring muscles lie at the back of the thigh. They comprise the semimembranosis, the semitendonosis, both on the inside of the thigh at the back, and the biceps femoris, which lies on the outside at the back. These three muscles are attached to the bottom of the pelvis at the back, and run down the back of the thigh to various points just below the knee. They are the main muscles that bend the knee, and hence are antagonistic to the quadriceps muscle. They are the bane of sprinters, and as soccer is a sprint recovery sport, hamstring injury and pain are an important cause of loss of pitch-time. The forces involved in hamstring disruption can be sufficient to cause avulsion fracture at the attachment of the muscle at the base of the pelvis. This is when part of the bone, where the muscle is attached, is pulled away, rather than the muscle itself being torn. It is more common in teenage players, where the growing part of the bone is softer.

During the act of sprinting the sudden straightening of the knee requires the lengthening of the hamstring to accommodate that movement. At the point of foot strike, there has to be a sudden, controlling, contraction of the hamstring muscle. This contraction is coordinated with the simultaneous contraction of the quadriceps muscle (at the front of the thigh). Obviously, without these contractions occurring, and being in tune with each other, the leg would give way, being unable to support the forces put through it.

During sprinting, as the hamstring is lengthening, the sudden superimposed contraction can cause disruption or tearing of the muscle. There are, of course, large forces put through the hamstrings at this time, and if

179

the muscle is weak and cannot withstand the contraction, it will give way, causing tearing. This can happen at any point in the muscle.

If the muscles are not coordinated properly, there may be a loss of synchronization of contraction during running. The time frames are too small in sprinting to allow for adjustment if the contractions are not well co-ordinated. Also, the forces are greater. This leaves the hamstring muscle open to disruption. Why should this happen?

It concerns neuro–muscular co-ordination, or the integration of muscle contraction with the nerve impulses received by the muscle, which is essential for normal movement. The hamstring muscles are supplied by nerve roots from the lower lumbar spine, and if they are irritated in any way, for instance by an intervertebral disc or an inflamed facet joint, this will interfere with the messages sent to, and received by, the hamstring muscle. This can lead to the muscle not contracting at exactly the right time, and becoming disrupted.

Also, if the muscle is not conditioned properly, or has not gone through a thorough rehabilitation after injury, it may not be strong or be able to respond to the normal nerve input necessary for the sudden contraction required in sprinting. Once again, this could easily lead to muscle disruption.

As the causes of hamstring injuries are multifactorial, an holistic approach to the injury must be taken.

In making a diagnosis, the case history is important. If there is a sudden tear, or an avulsion, the player will feel 'something go'. However, it is not uncommon for the player to experience tightening in the muscle. This may be due to a tear, but may be due to failure of neuro–muscular co-ordination: the messages from the nervous system to the muscle are not getting there at the right time, or are not being acted upon by the muscle. Hence, after taking a comprehensive case history, the medical team will exhaustively examine the lumbar area, pelvis, and hamstrings to try to gain some insight into the mechanism of injury. In the early stages of the injury, the root cause is not always obvious, and although a theory of cause can be put forward, it is important to be open to re-interpretation of the clinical picture as the injury and healing process evolve.

Imaging is helpful; X-ray examination will show an avulsion if it is present, while MRI scanning of both the hamstring and the lumbar spine area will help demonstrate the extent of any local disruption, and also whether there is any evidence of nerve pressure that could be responsible for the failure of co-ordination. Once again, ultrasound scanning in tandem with MRI will aid in more accurately determining the extent of any disruption, and hence prognosis and time to recovery.

Even if there is evidence of a disruption in the muscle, the cause may still be one associated with the lumbar spine. Occasionally, there appears to be no structural problem, but when nerve conduction studies are undertaken, to measure the nerve impulses sent to and received by the hamstrings, it is found that the nerve impulse is being interrupted. This test can pinpoint the site of nerve pressure, hence unlocking the difficult diagnostic problem that this type of injury can pose.

Treatment has to be targeted at the cause of the disruption. However, because of the intimate relationship between the lumbar spine and its nerve roots, and the hamstring muscles, rehabilitation must be co-ordinated between the two, as are the movement patterns in health.

The muscle disruption itself should be treated with manual physical therapy and electro-therapy as appropriate. Any neurological issues must be addressed at the same time. If there is a structural problem in the lumbar spine, this should be addressed. Facet joint inflammation can be alleviated with NSAIDs, or injection of steroid delivered under direct CT scan guidance. Similarly, if there is an intervertebral disc bulge, a caudal epidural injection might help. If these are ineffective, or there is another anatomical issue in the lumbar spine, for instance a spondylolisthesis, surgical intervention may be required. In the recreational footballer, this may be an extreme treatment for something which, over time, and with good physical therapy, will get better. However, for professional footballers, surgical intervention may be sought earlier, as time spent in rehabilitation has a risk of being time wasted if total alleviation of symptoms is not achieved.

The nature of the contraction of the hamstring in sprinting is eccentric. That is to say, the muscle lengthens as it contracts. Early in rehabilitation this type of contraction is essential, as the co-ordination repeatedly mentioned is integral in recurrence prevention. It also ensures that the new, regenerating, muscle fibres and scar tissue are laid down in the lines of force of the muscle–tendon unit. This means that the healed tissue will be more resilient when put under the forces encountered in sprinting.

Prevention is aided by attaining a good range of motion, in common with other muscle injuries. Imagine the kicking action: the hamstring group of muscles has to be flexible enough to accommodate this type of excursion. In the past, having longer

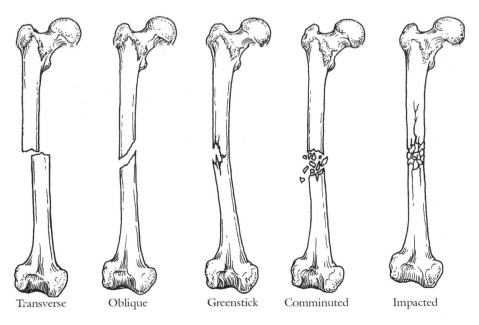

| Transverse | Oblique | Greenstick | Comminuted | Impacted |

Fractures of the femur.

hamstrings has been a 'holy grail of stretching' for athletes. However, current thinking is that strength and the learning of the co-ordination between the nervous system and the muscle are just as important, if not more so.

These three elements are essential in the prevention of hamstring injuries. What is also important is to look at the whole of the way the lumbar spine and pelvis move together. If there is a stiff area in the lumbar spine, perhaps from previous injury, or from acute, relatively minor, local trauma in a match, there may be less movement in this area, and more movement elsewhere, for example, in the pelvic region. If this is so, the hamstring will have to stretch more, thereby leaving the muscle group open to injury.

It is important therefore to take into account the rest of the musculo-skeletal system when considering hamstring rehabilitation and injury prevention. Of course, we have mentioned the importance of this type of approach before, but for the hamstrings the case is perhaps more important.

Fracture of the Femur

Fractures of the thighbone are rare in soccer. A fractured femur usually happens with a single blow but stress fractures are also possible in sports such as long distance running and triathlon (especially women with few or no periods). The stress fracture generally feels like a generalized pain in the thigh and will probably not be a sharp pain as it would be with a complete fracture. A number of fractures are possible, including a compound fracture.

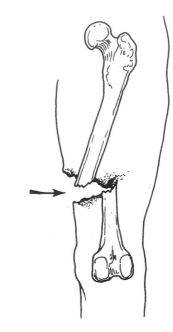

Compound fracture of the femur.

Self help for cramps

1 Break the cramp in the calf muscle by bending the ankle forward. It is best to have a second person break the cramp for you. For a hamstring cramp, lie on your back, flex the thigh up, let the other person forcefully push down on the ball of your foot to break the cramp.

2 Sometimes the cramp will reoccur shortly. Just repeat the procedure and massage the muscle to increase the circulation.

CHAPTER 20

Injuries to the Knee

The knee is the largest joint in the body. It is a synovial joint, with a joint capsule surrounding it, and comprises two parts: one between the thighbone and the shinbone (the tibio–femoral joint), and one between the thighbone and the knee-cap (the patello–femoral joint). Both have their particular problems.

The knee is a modified hinge joint. It is lined by the smooth membranous substance called hyaline cartilage, which helps to redistribute the forces experienced by the weight-bearing surfaces. Without this, the same areas of both bones would be loaded with each step taken, and damage from wear would be inevitable. The tibia or shinbone has a rather flat top, slightly asymmetrical. This is made into more of a cup by the menisci. These are made of fibro-cartilage and sit on the rims, both on the inside and outside, of the shinbone. They also act as shock absorbers, and are important in protecting the joint from degenerative disease.

The joint is supported by collateral ligaments, one on the inside (medial), and one on the outside (lateral). The medial ligament is a strong structure, helping to prevent a 'knock-

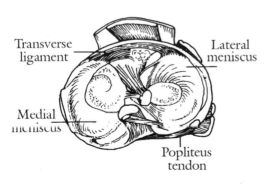

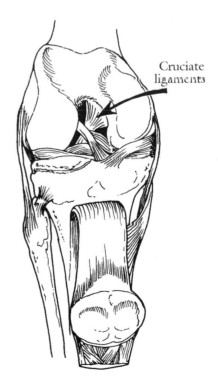

Top and front view of the knee.

kneed' injury, as well as helping to prevent a rotational injury. There are strong supporting structures at the back of the knee on the inside and on the outside which also lend support.

In the knee itself, there are two ligaments that cross over each other called the cruciate ligaments. One starts off at the front part of the shinbone and runs upwards and backwards to the thighbone. This is the anterior cruciate ligament (ACL). The other runs from the back part of the shinbone, and runs upwards and forwards to the thighbone. This is the posterior cruciate ligament (PCL). The cruciate ligaments prevent excessive front-to-back movement of the shin and thighbones upon each other. The ACL also helps to prevent excessive rotation of the thigh and shinbones on each other.

The knee-cap, or patella, is held in place partly by the tendon that is formed by the condensation of the quadriceps muscle into the patellar ligament or tendon, which inserts into the shinbone in the front near the top. The other stabilizers of the patella are the patello–femoral ligaments, between the knee-cap and the thighbone. These vary in the amount of movement they allow. The back of the knee-cap is lined with a thick layer of hyaline cartilage, the thickest anywhere in the body: the forces placed through this joint can be between three and six times body weight.

Many epidemiological studies over the years have shown that the knee and ankle are the most commonly injured joints in soccer.

KNEE INJURIES

The most useful way to approach this topic is to describe the way a new injury is presented to the coach or medical team. We will then discuss the structures, and finally we can address the problem of treatment and prevention.

Sudden Swelling

If the player sustains an injury and the joint swells within an hour, this indicates a haemarthrosis, that is to say there is bleeding into the joint. In 70% of these cases, the anterior cruciate ligament (ACL) will be ruptured. This ligament has a blood supply and the artery becomes damaged along with the ligament, resulting in bleeding. The player will often experience a pop or bang in the knee as the ligament ruptures, and this can be elicited when questioning the player prior to examination. The other causes of a knee haemarthrosis are:

- a capsular tear
- meniscal tears (usually at the periphery of the meniscus, and more commonly in young teenagers, as the meniscus has a rather more generous blood supply than is present in later life), and
- osteochondral fractures, where the trauma of an injury can disrupt the smooth membrane (the hyaline cartilage) along with the small piece of bone that it is attached to.

Delayed Swelling

If the swelling takes 12–24 hours to appear, this is more suggestive of a meniscus tear, but one which does not involve a part of the meniscus that has a blood supply. The other cause of this type of swelling is ligament disruption, or direct trauma causing bruising. The player will often say, 'when I woke up it was like a balloon'.

Locking

The knee is said to be locked when the normal range of motion is limited in extension. The player will experience an inability voluntarily to push the knee backwards when standing. The reason for this symptom is that something gets stuck in the joint. This is either a loose body, usually a piece of redundant bone, or a torn meniscus. When the meniscus is torn, a small scrap, which is sometimes called a 'parrot's beak', may become displaced and prevent the joint from straightening properly. It is like something being placed in the edge of a doorway, by the hinges, preventing the door from closing properly. The nature of this type of tear is that the scrap, or fragment, can easily become replaced in its normal position, until the next time it is jolted from position, when the knee will not straighten properly, and cause locking.

Giving Way

Sometimes the player will complain of the knee giving way. True giving way occurs without warning, with the player falling to the floor, sometimes with pain. Some players will have giving way, but will say that they felt pain, and it was this that caused the giving way. This is not 'true' giving way, and the cause for the pain must be sought first.

Giving way is caused by a loose body, which may, at an inappropriate time, become caught in the joint where it interferes with normal movement, and the joint is unable to attain a position where it can support one's body weight. A meniscal scrap, or remnant, could be the cause.

Giving way can also be caused by deficient ligament support. This usually means a deficient anterior cruciate ligament. The ACL prevents abnormal rotation of the tibia and femur on each other. The player may complain that as they cut from one line of running to another, in changing direction, the knee may give way without warning. In this on-field activity, the ACL has a unique function in relaying messages to the brain as to how much rotational force is going through the knee, and allows the adjustment of posture and muscle action to protect the joint and the surrounding tissue. Obviously, without the ACL, this reflex action is lost, and the knee gives way at the point of greatest shear, often resulting in damage to the weight-bearing surfaces in the joint.

Anterior Cruciate Ligament Rupture

The ACL's anatomy has already been described. It limits front-to-back movement of the tibia on the femur as well as limiting rotation of these two bones on each other. It does both these things by a mechanical restraint, the ligament itself, and by stimulating a reflex action of the muscles surrounding the knee (see 'giving way' above), enabling them to protect the joint. Its rupture is a major event in the life of a soccer player. In years past, it meant the end of a player's career, but in modern times, ACL reconstruction is practised worldwide, and very successfully. It allows players to return to play, even at the very highest level.

It still takes 6–12 months to return to play, depending on the extent of the injury, and the effectiveness of rehabilitation.

The cause of ACL rupture is often non-contact. It usually occurs when the player is changing direction, and the foot is misplaced. The normal ACL reflex action of the muscles is not quick enough to prevent overstretching of the ligament, and it ruptures, resulting in immediate swelling of the joint, often evident by the time the player has reached the medical room, but certainly in the next few hours.

Tackles causing a valgus (knock-kneed) stress on the joint may open the joint up enough to cause a similar injury to the ACL.

The diagnosis is made primarily from the case history. The player will often feel a pop in the knee, and say that the joint swelled quickly. Careful examination by the medical team may be painful, although not invariably, in the acute phase. The front–back translation of the thigh and shinbones should be compared with the other side. In ACL rupture, the affected side will show greater translation and confirm the suspicion. Beware, however, the posterior cruciate ligament injury. This will also show greater translation.

X-rays, especially in the younger player, may show a tearing off of the piece of bone on the top of the tibia to which the ACL is attached. This is unusual, however, and apart from identifying the obvious swelling, plain X-rays are usually unhelpful. MRI scanning has revolutionized the diagnosis of ACL rupture. It is also useful because the ACL is often injured as part of an injury complex, which can involve a meniscal tear, and other ligament damage. If this is the case, early recognition of the meniscal tear may mean this particular part of the problem can be surgically addressed early on, if deemed appropriate, and may result in a shorter recovery time.

Treatment of ACL rupture

The treatment depends on many issues, those concerning the injury itself but also the player's own situation. If the player is a professional, ACL reconstruction is carried out, usually after a wait of approximately six weeks. This delay is because the injury is a very traumatic and inflammatory event. The inflammation continues, even if the operation is carried out immediately, and can cause overwhelming scarring and ultimately constriction of the tissues surrounding the joint, causing restriction in motion.

In some countries, ACL reconstruction is more likely to be undertaken regardless of the level of the player. Some countries will rehabilitate the player, and if that fails, reconstruction then follows. There are arguments both for and against these two approaches. The research suggests that some players will be able to return to play without reconstruction. The ACL is a structure that has a dual role: it stops excessive movement mechanically, but also by the reflex action of muscles instigated by the stretching of the ligament itself. This ability to prevent abnormal movement around the knee that would cause dysfunction can be learnt by the other tissues (ligaments, capsule, muscle) around the joint. The conundrum is that we have no way of telling who may, or may not, be able to do this. In other words, players are sent to rehabilitation but, unusually, they embark upon this arduous task not knowing how things will turn out.

Medical personnel are used to dealing with uncertainty, but soccer players, in general, are not, and they are not that interested in the academic discussion surrounding this type of uncertainty. In this situation players may opt for a reconstruction even if they may have successfully rehabilitated without surgery. However, having the surgery does not exclude the player from the arduous rehabilitation afterwards.

Meniscal tears and ACL ruptures have some common symptoms: locking and giving way. A meniscal tear will be dealt with by arthroscoping the knee (keyhole surgery) soon after the injury. The normal course of management, outlined above, should then be pursued. This is where MRI is useful: dagnosing a meniscal tear will prevent the player rehabilitating for a knee that has another cause for giving way and swelling. If a knee with both these injuries is rehabilitated without the meniscal injury being addressed, the player may fail rehabilitation because of either the meniscal injury, the ACL rupture, or both. Dealing with the meniscal injury early saves time.

Despite the debate about the best management for this problem, the long-term outcome is usually the early onset of degenerative joint disease. This is thought to be due to the lack of co-ordinated fine movements in the joint, because of the loss of the fine tuning reflex action instigated by the ACL. This degeneration is made worse by any injury to the other structures in the joint at the same time as that to the ACL.

The only way to prevent ACL rupture is to have excellent proprioception with regard to the ACL. There is no doubt that this ligament is full of stretch receptors which send messages to the brain, and by reflex action cause muscles to contract and relax in a concerted way in order to protect the joint.

This is done by mimicking game situations as much as possible. This should preferably be carried out on the field of play, but can be

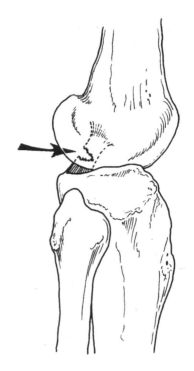

Anterior cruciate ligament tear.

done, especially during rehabilitation, in the gymnasium.

Posterior Cruciate Ligament Injury

The PCL starts at the back of the top, or plateau, of the tibia and runs upwards and forwards to attach to the femur. Its function is to prevent excessive backward movement of the tibia with regard to the femur. It works in concord with some structures at the back, and on the outside part, of the knee. These structures are given the collective name of the 'postero-lateral corner'. That is to say, the structures are at the outside back corner of the knee. Together they help prevent rotational injuries, not unlike the ACL. They comprise mainly a large tendon from the popliteus muscle, and the lateral collateral ligament (LCL).

The classic PCL injury, called the 'dashboard injury', is caused by sitting in the passenger seat of a car involved in a road traffic accident. The bent knee bangs up against the dashboard, forcing the shinbone backwards, causing the PCL to rupture. In soccer, this is a contact injury. When a player has a knee that is bent to 90°, and an opponent runs into the tibia, it can fracture, but if the trauma is directed at the upper part of the shinbone, the result is more likely to be a PCL rupture.

As with the ACL, the other structures associated with this type of injury can be more important. When the PCL is injured the postero-lateral structures are often injured at the same time. This is especially so with trauma that causes backward movement of the tibia, as well as opening up the outside of the joint, causing tearing of these structures. It is this injury complex that causes instability. An isolated PCL tear does not cause giving way, but a postero-lateral corner disruption can, and hence can become much more of a management problem.

In terms of diagnosis, the pain will be too great for the player to be examined soon after the injury, so the usual first aid must be applied. The PCL rupture can be identified by demonstrating the increased back-to-front movement of the tibia on the mur. This time though, it is the backward movement of the tibia that is more evident. This can sometimes be difficult to see, but can be demonstrated by lying the player on a couch, bending both knees up to about 60°, and then looking from the side. As you follow the edge of the shinbone up, over the knee-cap, the profile is a convex one. The PCL injured side will show a concave profile, demonstrating the shinbone falling backwards. At this time, it is easier to appreciate the 'dashboard injury'. The postero-lateral corner must always be carefully assessed to make sure that it is not also injured.

X-rays may show if there is an injured bone. Stress views can be carried out. This is when the knee is held in a position that will demonstrate any laxity, and an X-ray taken. However, MRI scanning is now the mainstay of investigation in this type of injury, which can be difficult to manage. The scan will show a swollen disrupted PCL, and will give valuable insight into the extent of the postero-lateral corner damage, should there be any. This allows a more accurate stab at prognosis.

An isolated PCL injury will need physiotherapy and rehabilitation, and may take a player two to three months to recover from; reconstruction is not usually recommended. Reconstruction is carried out, but the improvement in symptoms may not be enough to outweigh the risks of surgery. Rehabilitation should make sure that the restraining action of the quadriceps is strong enough to compensate for the lack of a PCL to maintain the shinbone in the right place. This process should go on throughout a playing career so that the muscles do not gradually deteriorate. After the loss of the PCL, the knee's synchronized motion changes subtly so that, over time, degenerative change becomes more likely.

With postero-lateral corner injury, surgery is much more likely to improve the stability of the knee. If both injuries are present, surgery is often undertaken on the postero-lateral corner first, with PCL surgery being offered later, when reassessment of the joint after the initial surgery is possible.

Medial Collateral Ligament Injuries

The MCL is situated on the inside of the knee, and is attached to the femur (thighbone) and the tibia (shinbone). It runs quite a long way down onto the inside of the tibia, and as it does so, runs slightly forwards. The textbooks say it attaches to the tibia a 'hands breadth' below the line of the knee joint (where the two bones meet).

This very strong ligament has two main functions:

• to stop the knee becoming too 'knock-kneed' when a tackle is made to the outside of the knee: the MCL stops the knee from opening up on the inside

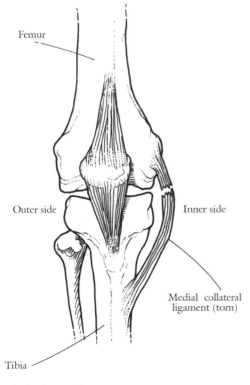

Medial collateral ligament tear.

• to aid the ACL in preventing too much rotation of the tibia on the femur; this is why the ligament runs slightly forwards, as well as downwards.

There are three grades of tear, in line with the grading for muscle, ligament and tendon injuries described in Chapter 3.

The cause of MCL tears is usually traumatic. A tackle from the side of the player may transmit a force across the knee joint from outside to inside. The MCL resists this force, together with the muscles and other tissues on the inside of the joint. If the force is great enough, tearing of the ligament, and sometimes the other tissues involved in restraint will occur. If the knee is bent on impact, and the foot is on the floor, the MCL is isolated and is more vulnerable than if the knee is fully straightened, when the other tissues help resist the force.

Diagnosis is made by the medical team of physiotherapists and doctors who will have noted the case history, and will be able to examine the knee carefully. This injury is very painful, and examination just after the injury may not be of much help, as the extent may be impossible to ascertain. In some players the MCL may be lax anyway. This can be because both knees have normally lax ligaments, an anatomical variation from normal. The other cause is that the MCL may have been injured in the past. It is important then, that both knees should be evaluated and compared.

Plain X-rays are helpful in the case of the rare avulsion fracture, but ultrasound and MRI scans are the mainstay of radiological investigation for this type of injury. In severe cases of MCL tears, the ACL and menisci are vulnerable, and are evident on MRI scan.

Treatment depends on the severity of

189

the injury. The research literature is full of studies comparing surgical and non-surgical treatment but, in general, Grade I and minor Grade II injuries are managed non-surgically with physiotherapy and rehabilitation. Higher Grade II tears are put in a brace for six weeks with a limitation on the range of motion. Still higher Grade II and Grade III tears may be treated surgically. Obviously, whether there are other structures involved in the injury will have a bearing on recourse to surgical intervention.

Prevention is partly about the rules of the game. The more harsh the punishment for tackles that cause this type of injury, the lower the incidence will be. Accidents will happen, but over the years, rule changes about tackling have reduced the severity of this injury.

Lateral Collateral Ligament Injury

The lateral collateral ligament does a similar job to the MCL, but on the outside of the joint. It prevents the knee becoming too 'bow-legged'. That is to say that it stops the outside of the knee joint opening up. It is not as strong as the MCL, nor as long. When sitting in a cross-legged position, it can be felt by running the fingers along the joint line between the femur and tibia, and feels like a cord. This is the LCL.

It does not need to be as strong, because it has support from the other, very strong, structures that form the postero-lateral corner. These structures act in unison, but if the postero-lateral structures are involved in the injury, an unstable knee is often the result.

As with the MCL, these injuries are caused by trauma, usually in a tackle. If a player goes to kick the ball, and the opponent's foot makes contact with the upper tibia, the foot may follow through, and the knee open up on the outside, causing tearing of the structures on the outside.

The difficulty with diagnosing injuries to the outside of the knee is deciding to what extent the other structures are involved. Injuries to the lateral side of the knee joint can involve the LCL, the popliteus tendon, the joint capsule, the lateral hamstrings and PCL.

Accurate examination may take a few days, as the injury is a painful one. This is, once again, where MRI scanning can help judge the extent of the injury. It may not change what happens in the first days of an injury, but it may help plan treatment. The player also then has an idea of what the injury actually is.

Once again, when examining, the other knee should be assessed first, so that the 'normal' situation can be compared with the injured knee.

Treatment depends on the extent of the other structures' involvement. If the postero-lateral corner opens up to any degree when examined, this will almost certainly mean that the player will need a reconstruction of this area. In less severe injuries, the player may rehabilitate after a period of physical therapy. However, if the knee is unstable, early surgery is advised, as the torn postero-lateral structures scar, contract, and are less easy to reassemble.

Meniscal Tears

There are two menisci (singular = meniscus). They sit on the top (plateau) of the tibia, and run around the rim, one on the inside and

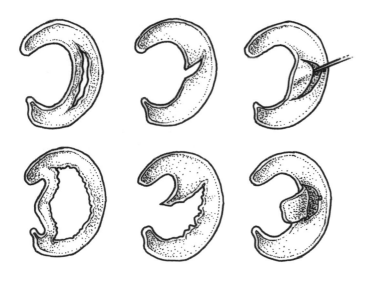

Types of meniscal tear.

one on the outside. They are attached to the tibia on their outer edges by small but strong ligaments. They act to make the relatively flat top of the tibia more of a cup, to receive the rounded femur. They also act as important shock absorbers for the knee joint. They are sometimes called the semi-lunar cartilages, perhaps a more comprehensible term. They are made of a strong fibrous tissue, akin to gristle.

Different types of tear can occur and there have been attempts at a classification in order to allow better prediction of outcome after surgery. In soccer, the inside (medial) meniscus is more commonly injured.

The cause of the injury is clear. In soccer, cleats, or studs, are attached to the sole of the boot to aid grip. The meniscus, like most other structures in and around the knee, is susceptible to twisting forces. This is especially so when the knee is bent, and the thigh and calf have some degree of independence in the amount each part may twist. When the knee is extended, and the leg is straight, the calf follows what the thigh does, giving the knee more, but not absolute, protection.

The classic way the meniscus is torn is when the foot is fixed on the turf, the knee is bent, and the thigh twists on the knee when weight is borne through the joint. The player often feels a tearing sensation, and obviously has pain. The player may try to continue, but is often unable to. Players usually say that the knee was painful, did not swell straight away, but by the evening or the following morning it was like a balloon.

There are many other ways in which the meniscus is injured. The biomechanical make-up of the player has some effect on the vulnerability of the meniscus. Players often have 'bow-legs', and this can cause nipping of the inner part of the meniscus that sits on the inside of the knee.

The meniscus on the outside can be torn in such a way that a cyst forms on it. This is much more common than with the inside meniscus. The cyst usually becomes more painful and prominent after exercise, as it fills with fluid. The cyst is there because there is a horizontal tear in the meniscus itself, and fluid creeps through this during exercise, causing the swelling.

Rarely, during development, the meniscus may not form properly and is left misshapen, like a disc. This is known as a discoid meniscus, and usually occurs in the outside, or lateral, meniscus. It is noteworthy as it can be torn more easily than the normal meniscus. As you can imagine, the disc-like structure can more easily become trapped between the bones of the femur and tibia.

In diagnosis, the medical team will take a careful history of how the injury occurred. If they were present, they may have seen the incident. A careful examination will follow. The knee will probably be swollen, and there may be difficulty in straightening it. This is known as 'locking'. The menisci themselves cannot be felt, but the areas around the joint line may be tender when pressed. By this, we mean that with the player lying on their back on the couch, with the knee bent, the rim of the top of the shinbone can be felt; this is the joint line, and if feeling around it gives pain, this is indicative of a meniscal tear.

If the meniscus is disrupted or torn, there will be nothing to see on X-ray, but MRI scan will usually show the tear, which looks like a small white line going through the usually homogeneously black meniscus.

The treatment of this injury has changed radically in the last thirty years or so. Before the days of MRI scans, the diagnosis was made clinically only, often delayed as treatment by way of physiotherapy was attempted first. This was reasonable, as opening the knee at an operation and taking out the meniscus was the standard treatment. Arthroscopy, or keyhole surgery, changed this approach,

as the meniscus could be seen much easier, and the extent of the damage assessed more accurately. This meant that new instruments developed in tandem, and their use meant that the extent of surgery on the meniscus could be reduced, and at least part of it could be preserved. Nowadays, surgeons can, in certain circumstances, repair a meniscus. This is more rewarding if the player is pre-pubertal or if the player has ample blood supply to the injured part of the meniscus. With ageing, the blood supply retreats to the periphery, making repair less successful.

The problem with having had a meniscus removed is that the buffering effect is lost, and degenerative changes inevitably follow. After operative intervention, it is always important for the player to enter a rehabilitation programme to make sure that the muscles around the joint are strong again, and also that the proprioception related to the joint is back to normal.

As far as prevention goes, there is no doubt that footwear, surface conditions, and bad luck have a part to play in meniscal injuries. However, if the proprioception of the joint is optimal, the twisting injuries may be avoided by the reflex action of hanging posture and weight distribution during a manoeuvre. Strapping and bracing may help prevent the twisting, but there is, at the moment, no real evidence to prove this, and in a contact sport anti-rotation braces may be deemed dangerous.

Osgood–Schlatter Disease

This is not a disease, but was originally described as such, and the name has stuck.

Whilst the skeleton is still growing, the area of bone that is actively laying down new bone is softer than normal. With the long bones, like the shinbone, new bone is laid down in layers, one on top of the other. The layers are not distinguishable: the new bone integrates with the bone already there. The tibia has a large tendon attached to it just below the knee joint at the front of the bone. During the time that the player is growing, this attachment is an area of softer bone like that mentioned above. In footballers, usually in mid-teens, this softer bone is pulled upon by the tendon that attaches to it, which is the quadriceps tendon. With repetitive traction the soft bone becomes inflamed and painful. This is Osgood–Schlatter disease. It is often found on one side only, usually the dominant, or kicking leg (*see* diagram on p. 26).

This is an overuse injury, caused by kicking, running and jumping. The amount of play causing this varies in each individual, as each player grows at a slightly different rate, and hits their growth spurt at a certain time, usually different from other team-mates.

Diagnosis is made by listening to the player, and doing a careful examination. The player will say that the more they play, the worse it gets. Pain will invariably follow exercise. If the area at the front of the knee is felt, there will be some pain and swelling. X-rays in this age group should be avoided if possible, as the young growing skeleton is more susceptible to radiation effects. There is, on occasion, pressure from parents to have an X-ray, but if the player rests for a few weeks and everything settles, this may be avoided. Equally, if things do not settle, and the player is truthful about the amount of rest taken, then an X-ray is probably reasonable.

There is no real treatment for this problem except rest. Despite rest, some players have very troublesome pain for many months before it settles completely. The usual scenario is that, after rest for 4–6 weeks, the player can gently return to training and playing. Talented young players are often asked to play many games in a season, as they are wanted by various teams. However, care must be taken with these players. The consequence of over-playing is no playing at all because of overuse injuries.

Treatment really amounts to secondary prevention. As the bones grow, especially in the growth spurt, the muscles lengthen slower than the bones, so causing a pulling on the tendon attachment by the muscles being shorter. This is compounded by the repetitive action of kicking. Bear in mind that, at this stage of growth, the muscles are becoming stronger and will therefore be more forceful.

To prevent this injury it is therefore very important to make sure that all the muscle groups that attach around the knee are stretched. This includes the quadriceps, the hamstrings and the calf muscles. Primary prevention should be attempted, and a graded stretching programme, anticipating the growth spurt, should be instigated.

Patellar Tendonopathy

Patellar tendonopathy describes a syndrome that causes pain in the tendon, almost invariably around the point where the tendon and patella meet. The patellar tendon is the structure by which the knee straightens. When the quadriceps muscle contracts, it pulls on the patellar tendon, which then pulls on the shinbone, causing the leg to straighten. This tendon is a large structure, transmitting large forces, up to twelve times body weight during slow extension, and up to nine times body weight during fast extension. The latter is what one might expect more commonly in soccer. If you sit with your knee bent, and run your fingers over the knee-cap, or patella, going downwards, the patellar tendon can be felt as the thick structure joining the bottom of the patella to the shinbone. There has been much debate over the years about the cause of patellar tendon pain, because patellar tendonopathy has often proved difficult to treat.

Patellar tendonopathy is seen more commonly in sports where persistent jumping is part of the game. Basketball and volleyball are two such sports. It is not uncommon in soccer, and is not confined to players from one position.

Originally, it was thought that there was inflammation in the tendon, or between it and the tendon sheath. However, the absence of the cells and chemicals that are markers of inflammation in the body has caused us to re-think what is going on microscopically. This is why the name patellar tendonopathy (diseased tendon), rather than tendonitis (inflamed tendon) is used. This has also meant a re-think on the treatment.

The cause of patellar tendon problems is complex. Biomechanical issues play a part, and foot type, posture and gait pattern can have a bearing on the origin of this problem. The leg should, more or less, move in a straight vertical line when walking or running, so if the foot rolls too much either in or out, or the pelvic and abdominal musculature cannot help hold the leg straight, the patellar tendon may suffer unequal stresses across it, causing tendon dysfunction.

Foot mechanics are important, but it should be remembered that core stability (pelvic and abdominal) also has a bearing on the way the lower limb works during exercise, and poor stability has consequences, often focused on the patellar tendon.

Overloading the tendon is another cause. For instance, asking players to run on hard ground, especially if the increase to a different intensity of training is sudden, can cause patellar tendon pain. This is also the case with gymnasium-based programmes.

Diagnosis is by examination and scanning. When felt, the tendon is often slightly thicker (wider), and is tender when the lower part of the patella is felt. X-ray will be unhelpful, unless there is a small amount of calcium in the tendon, such as new bone, which can be found on occasion. The mainstay of investigation is to ultrasound, or MRI scan the tendon. Ultrasound is probably the most helpful, as there are some changes in the tendon that are best seen with ultrasound.

The treatment is based around halting the progress of the syndrome, and reversing the changes in the tendon. First aid involves rest in this case. Icing might help with pain, but may have little effect on the process itself. After this initial period, which will vary depending on severity, a programme of eccentric training rehabilitation should be instigated. An eccentric muscle contraction is when a muscle is contracting and lengthening at the same time (see Chapter 12 for a more complete description and analysis). In a biceps curl, for example, the muscle shortens as the weight is lifted. This is a concentric contraction. As the weight is lowered, the muscle is still contracting, but lengthening. This is an eccentric contraction. This type of contraction puts more force through the muscle.

Eccentric training rehabilitation is a relatively new treatment, but is very successful. For those resistant to this type of treatment, injection therapy may be helpful. Lastly, surgery is a possibility. Before eccentric training rehabilitation, surgery for this complaint was much more common.

Prevention is often secondary, that is, instigated after the event, to prevent recurrence. Prevention before the event should start by making sure that core stability is of a good standard. Foot mechanics and type should be noted, but the prescription of orthotics to change the way the foot works before the onset of symptoms is very controversial. However, with information about the normal mechanical make-up of the player, orthotic prescription, if deemed appropriate, can be initiated. Care with new training programmes, making sure that increments are not too big, and that conditions are appropriate, will prevent the onset of this troublesome problem.

CHAPTER 21

Injuries to the Lower Leg

EXERCISE-RELATED LOWER LIMB PAIN

Exercise-related lower limb pain (ERLLP) has traditionally been called 'shin splints', but this may be more a symptom than a syndrome or disease process. Pain in the shin area or calf occurs when the player runs. Often the site of the pain is ill defined, but sometimes almost pinpointed. The pain can come on immediately when the player starts to run, or some time during the run. It may be relieved immediately when the player stops running, or persist for a day afterwards. The main three causes of ERLLP are:

1. Medial tibial stress syndrome (MTSS) or periostitis
2. Stress fracture of tibia or fibula
3. Compartment syndrome.

Causes of ERLLP

The biomechanics of a player may predispose to any of the three main causes. This bio-mechanical make-up would include central stability, foot posture, running style, musculature, flexibility, leg length, and many other factors. A certain training and playing regimen will result in an overuse injury in some players, while others may fare well, and be injury-free.

MTSS or periostitis

On the inside of the tibia (shinbone) are attached muscles that take part in the act of walking and running. These are the plantar flexors, and when contracted the toes point downwards. The muscles condense into tendons that are attached to the bones in the foot and the toes. As they contract, they pull on the toes to allow movement, while at the other end the muscle pulls on the edge of the tibia. Around all bones is a structure called the periosteum (*peri* = around, and *osteum* = bone). This structure is like a membrane, and is very sensitive to trauma of any kind. If the muscle pulls excessively on the periosteum, it becomes inflamed and painful. Periostitis causes pain that comes on during exercising, and can last a day or so after stopping exercise.

The primary cause of this complaint is overuse, especially in younger players who have often just recently joined a team or club. The step up from recreational football to playing and training regularly can put great strains on the growing musculo-skeletal system. Over-pronation of the foot while running is a common cause. In the action of running, the foot often rolls inwards, and the arch of the foot flattens. Pronation is a part of the normal gait cycle, but some players over-pronate. This pulls on the tendons that run around the ankle bone on the inside and, in turn, this pulls on the edge of the tibia where the muscles are. This irritates the periosteum that covers the bone, causing pain. The classical site for the pain is on the inside of the shinbone, usually about a third of the way up the bone.

Stress fracture

A stress fracture begins as a hairline crack in the bone. During the act of running, the two bones in the lower leg (the tibia and fibula) move together. The muscles on these two bones are trying to pull the bones the other way during the same action of running, thereby causing a shearing stress in the bone. The bone starts to crack. At first this is microscopic, but can convert to a full fracture if the activity continues. This pain begins as soon as the player starts to run. The classical description is 'crescendo pain': the pain gets worse and worse with exercise, until the player has to stop. The pain can carry on for a few hours after stopping running.

Stress fractures occur in very similar circumstances to MTSS. Much of the research about stress fractures of the lower limb in young people has been done on military recruits. It was noticed that a step-up in training, and in the case of soccer, playing, can cause stress reactions in the tibia and fibula.

It may be that, in some cases, stress fractures are just an extension in severity of MTSS: some players might play with MTSS and progress to stress fracture. However, there is no doubt that some players present with stress fractures without having previously had MTSS.

Compartment syndrome

The muscles in the leg operate in compartments. There are four of these in the leg between the knee and the ankle. They enclose the muscles in a fibrous material called 'fascia', rather like a plastic bag except that it is not inert like plastic, but can expand.

During exercise, the blood supply to the muscles is increased, allowing nutrients and oxygen to enter the muscle, thereby allowing the continuation of exercise. When the blood supply to a muscle increases, its volume will increase. However, in some players, the muscles may swell too much, and the fascia covering the muscle cannot expand sufficiently to accommodate this. In this situation, the pressure in the compartment increases until it exceeds the pressure of blood coming in. The muscle now has to exercise without any oxygen or fuel, and cramp-like pains begin. The pain disappears almost immediately after stopping running. Then the pressure inside the compartment falls and the by-products of exercise are quickly flushed through the muscle, and as normality returns, the pain subsides.

The cause of compartment syndrome may have a biomechanical basis, but the picture regarding cause in this situation is more hazy. It may be that some players have a fascia that is less able to accommodate the expansion. Or, that with excessive training, micro-trauma to the fascia causes some minor scarring, reducing the ability of the fascia to expand when required. It may be that the muscle simply grows too big for its compartment with training.

Diagnosis of ERLLP

Taking an accurate story from the player as to how the injury started, when the pain comes on during exercise, and when it goes, should point the medical team to a diagnosis. Examination is usually confirmatory. In MTSS and stress fractures of the tibia, the inside of this bone is tender as the physiotherapist or physician runs their fingers up the inside edge of the bone. Stress fractures also display tenderness when the bone is pressed, tapped, or a vibrating tuning fork is placed on the skin over the most tender area. The fibula, although suffering stress fractures less often, shows the same findings. There is often nothing to find on examination of compartment syndrome. The diagnosis is made here with the case history, and by measuring the compartment pressures directly using pressure transducers connected to a pressure reading device that prints out the recordings.

In stress fractures and MTSS, X-rays may show some changes and even a crack in the bone in stress fractures, but this may not be the case, especially early on in the injury, such as during the first week. The most accurate way of diagnosing MTSS and stress fractures is by an isotope bone scan. The only problem is that it is a slightly inconvenient test to undergo. The player must attend for a small injection of radio-isotope, then be scanned. They have to return after three hours to be re-scanned. MRI scan is gaining more converts, and it is hoped the expense will come down, and make this more accessible.

Treatment of ERLLP

For MTSS and stress fractures, the treatment is rest. This does not have to be absolute, but to avoid further irritation, any exercise must be carefully monitored. Non-weight-bearing activity can be undertaken to allow the player to keep fit, such as aerobic and interval training that can be done in the pool or on a cycle. Stress fractures usually take 4–6 weeks to heal in the fibula, and 6–8 weeks in the tibia. MTSS can be less predictable, and can take anywhere from two to ten weeks to settle. Pulsed ultrasound to the area may reduce the pain of stress fractures. During the recovery period the player should make sure to maintain flexibility, both in the calf area and generally.

Any biomechanical issues can be addressed at relative leisure during this time. Central abdominal (core) stability should be as good as the player can manage. A podiatrist should assess the player's gait and running style with the aid of video analysis, and prescribe foot orthoses should they be deemed necessary.

In a small number of cases of MTSS, surgery may be indicated as a last resort. This is done to alleviate the excessive pulling on the bone. It is very effective and has a short recovery period, the player being able to run ten days or so after the operation.

In the more unusual case of stress fractures at the front of the tibia, surgery may be necessary. This takes the form of insertion of metal pins in the central cavity of the bone and prevents excessive movement of the bone when running, thereby reducing the stresses at the front edge.

The treatment for compartment syndrome is surgery. The fascia enveloping the compartment is split, allowing the muscle to expand as required.

Prevention of ERLLP

There is controversy on this issue. Some advocate biomechanical assessment and prescription of orthotic devices for shoes if it is judged that the player may develop problems. It may be that if the player is assessed bio-mechanically it would be possible to inter-vene earlier, avoiding an established disease process. There is debate about both of these approaches. With more modern techniques of measuring the forces encountered in running, it may be possible in the future to predict more accurately which players may 'run into' problems.

In professional soccer these problems usually start when young players join, and there is a big step-up in training. Therefore, most clubs now give these players a training programme to follow in the lead-up to joining.

There is some research evidence that track and field athletes who had played ball games early in life were somewhat protected from stress reactions later in their athletic careers. There has also been some research that shows that weak and uncoordinated muscu-lature around the hip can be associated with this type of injury. Shock absorbency, using cushioned insoles, has also been shown to be helpful in prevention.

From this emerging information, it is clear that it is possible to predict who is more liable to encounter ERLLP. Care should be taken in obtaining an exercise history, as well as a detailed assessment of the mechanics of running both as concerns the hip and pelvis, and the foot and ankle.

CALF INJURIES

The calf has two major muscles. They are the gas-trocnemius and the soleus. The gastrocnemius starts above the knee, at the back of the femur. The soleus starts just below the knee joint, at the back of the tibia. They both run down the calf and join to form the Achilles tendon, which attaches to the heelbone, or calcaneum.

Calf Strain or Tear

These injuries can occur at any time, but do occur more often after the age of thirty in soccer players. The reason for this is not clear, but recovery and rehabilitation can take longer in this age group.

Acute tears occur in jumping, springing off to sprint, and changing direction, in fact in any explosive action. Tears occur more often after previous injury, either to the calf, return-ing too early after injury, or the ankle, when the calf becomes shorter, stiffer, and slightly wasted after disuse during recovery.

When the calf is recurrently torn, biome-chanical issues may have a part to play. Foot posture and gait pattern and leg length differ-ences may be part of the picture.

The player usually feels acute pain in the calf and has to stop playing. Some may try to carry on, but players cannot run these injuries off and should be substituted. Playing on will only make the injury worse and prolong the time to recovery.

The road to diagnosis, as always, starts with the case history. After this, examina-tion will involve asking the player to stand on tiptoe, if they can, and a close inspection of the injured area. With the player lying face down, forcing the toes upwards with the knee bent, then straight, will determine which of the main calf muscles is involved. With the knee bent, the soleus is the muscle on stretch when the toes are forced upwards towards the shin. With the knee straight-ened, the gastrocnemius is the main muscle stretched.

Imaging with ultrasound and MRI will help to judge the extent of the damage, and give a more accurate idea of time to recovery. In a longstanding or recurrent calf injury, MRI may be useful to exclude occult disease (which is very rare), and the extent of scar build-up.

The treatment is the same as for any other muscle disruption. In the initial phase, the normal PRICE regimen should be adopted. After 48 hours, stretching and gentle eccentric exercise can be commenced. Non-steroidal anti-inflammatories may be useful at this stage, but the need should be assessed by the team physician. When the player has a full, painless stretch (*see* Screening on p. 42), more intense concentric and eccentric exercise can be instituted. After this phase the player will be able to run, first in straight lines, then zig-zagging, or cutting. They then use the ball and progress back into training and playing.

Flexibility and conditioning are important in the prevention of this injury. The muscle group should be kept as long as possible, so that at extremes of range of motion the muscle tendon unit is not over-stretched. Strength and proprioception are just as important. It is well known that muscles are essential shock-absorbers, and therefore conditioning in this way is important in injury prevention.

Achilles Tendon Injury

There is great debate at present about disease of the Achilles tendon, not unlike that surrounding patellar tendon disease. The Achilles tendon is formed from the condensation of the gastrocnemius and soleus muscles, and is attached to the heelbone, or calcaneum. It is used by the body to effect plantar flexion: the action of pointing the toes down towards the ground. There are various types of such tendon injury.

Tendon rupture

This is a notorious injury, which occurs without warning. The player classically feels as if they have been kicked from behind, and will often accuse a player next to them. The rupture will be felt as a pop or snap, and the sound may be audible from some distance.

Explosive movements are often responsible for this injury. Springing off from a standstill to sprint can cause excessive force through the tendon, reaching the point where the muscle–

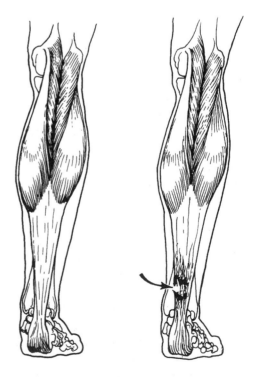

Achilles tendon and rupture.

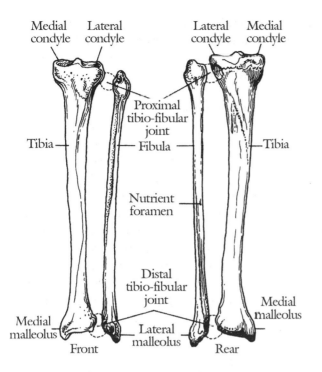

Medial condyle   Lateral condyle   Lateral condyle   Medial condyle

Proximal tibio-fibular joint

Tibia   Fibula   Tibia

Nutrient foramen

Distal tibio-fibular joint

Medial malleolus

Medial malleolus   Lateral malleolus

Front   Rear

The lower leg bones: tibia and fibula.

tendon unit is unable to absorb the energy produced, causing rupture. Typically a player lands from a jump, with the toes pointing downwards, and tries to sprint off immediately. By doing this, the muscle–tendon unit needs to stretch as the player lands, but the muscle contracts to begin the running motion. The tendon is therefore caught between stretch and contraction, causing excessive strain in the tendon, leading to rupture. There is some research evidence to suggest that if there is some tendon damage anyway, this predisposes to this type of injury.

The history of the injury is of paramount importance in diagnosis. The definitive examination test is performed with the player lying face down on the bench. The non-injured calf is squeezed in the middle of the calf. The toes point downwards. On the affected side, the toes remain still. The connection between the muscle and the heel has been severed, so the foot remains in the same posture. There is often a gap in the tendon itself, which the finger of the examiner can easily feel. If there is a lot of bleeding in the area, this may not be so obvious to the inexperienced.

Treatment is commonly surgery. The tendon is repaired and, in the early stages after surgery, the tendon is kept still in a cast to allow healing. Non-surgical treatment involves placing the foot in a cast, with the toes pointing downwards, which has been shown to have a similar outcome in Achilles tendon rupture. In professional soccer, the surgical approach is invariably used.

Rehabilitation after cast removal is based around flexibility and conditioning, but is slower than, for instance, a calf tear, although the same in principle. The rehabilitation is long, and it can take up to year before the player is back to playing properly.

Prevention is effected by flexibility and conditioning, although it cannot be prevented absolutely. Making sure that the tendon is healthy can also lessen the likelihood of rupture.

LOWER LEG FRACTURE

While shin guards are expected to reduce the number and severity of lower leg fractures, 90% of those suffering from lower leg fractures were wearing shin guards at the time of the trauma, and in 62% of the cases the contact which caused the fracture was to the shin guard. Tackles, particularly being tackled, are the major cause of this injury. Weaker bones, such as caused by the female athlete triad (*see* Chapter 23), can predispose to this injury.

Since a lower leg fracture to the tibia or fibula can vary from merely a crack to a compound fracture, X-rays are generally needed to determine its exact placement and severity.

While palpation of the bone or bones may be sufficient to determine that there is an injury, it may not be sufficient to determine its severity. Obviously proper setting and casting should be done as soon as practical.

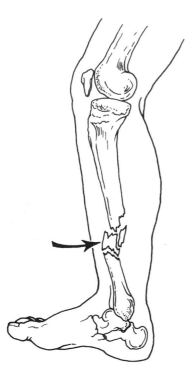

A serious fracture of the tibia.

Self help for shin splints

1   PRICE: use ice cup massage.

2   Strengthen the muscle by moving your foot upward against the pressure of your hand.

3   Wear full orthotics or arch supports (orthotics) or better cushioned shoes, or both. Commercial shoe inserts should also help.

4   Don't expect shin splints to heal themselves. They will get worse if you don't correct the problem.

5   If the problem is caused by running, run on soft sand or soft grass rather than a hard track or roadway.

CHAPTER 22

Injuries to the Ankle and Foot

Ankle sprains are certainly the most common injuries in soccer, accounting for lost playing time at all levels. The basic regime of ice, elevation and compression is followed for most ankle sprains, and a splint and crutches may be required for several days. However, the trend has been away from strict immobilization, even following severe sprains, and toward allowing the patient to begin as much weight bearing as can be tolerated and maintaining and increasing the ankle's range of motion.

Most soccer players will sustain numerous subungual hematomas of the toes during their career. These injuries generally occur to the great toe as the result of a direct crush by the foot of another player or from the shear stresses of sudden stops and starts as the toe impacts against the close-fitting toe box of the soccer cleat. For many players the toenail becomes dystrophic as the result of repeated

damage to the nailbed. Although seldom a serious problem, it can become troublesome.

THE ANKLE

The ankle is a complicated joint. It consists of the two long bones in the lower leg holding the talus in a swing joint. The talus is an unusual bone, as it is shaped in such a way as to help transmit forces from the vertical (the leg) to the horizontal (the foot). It is held in the 'vice' of the tibia and fibula by ligaments on the inside and the outside. The ones on the inside of the ankle are much stronger than those on the outside. The inside one is a single-layered, thick band of tissue that runs along the area between the tibia and the talus. The outside ligament complex is less strong and consists of three bands, one at the front,

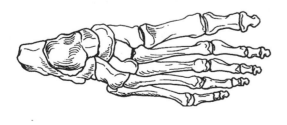

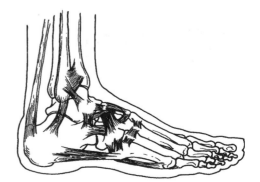

The ankle and foot bones and ligaments.

one in the middle and one at the back of the joint. The joint, which has a large capsule, is crossed on both sides, and in front, with the tendons that arise from the muscles that cause movements to the ankle, foot and toes. At the back is the Achilles tendon, and a pad of fat lies in front of this. In about 10% of people there is a small extra piece of bone at the back of the joint. This is called the os trigonum, and is important as it sometimes gets between the back of the tibia and the calcaneum, or heelbone, if the foot is forced into pointing downwards, for instance during a tackle.

ANKLE INJURIES

The ankle is the most commonly injured joint in soccer, accounting for about 25% of all soccer-related injuries presenting to accident and emergency departments. Of these, 80–90% are to the lateral ligaments. Any ankle injury with accompanied swelling should be X-rayed and evaluated by a doctor. Usually a specialist should be consulted as these injuries are often under-treated.

Ankle Sprain or Twist, and Ligament Disruption

The position and anatomy of the ankle make the ligaments around it prone to injury. The most commonly injured ligaments are the three on the outside.

An ankle sprain usually occurs with an 'inversion' injury, where the ankle twists inwards, so that the sole of the foot faces the other foot. The outside of the ankle is inherently more vulnerable because of its anatomy and because the outside ligaments are not as strong. The inside ligament of the ankle is less likely to be injured, but it makes a more serious injury.

The ligaments that join the two ankle bones just above the joint itself can also be injured. This can be serious, as the joint itself will be loosened. These ligaments are usually injured as part of a wider injury, generally a fracture of either or both of the ankle bones.

Sprains are caused by contact and non-contact situations during playing and training. The player may be running, and hit a small divot in the turf. The ankle will twist inwards,

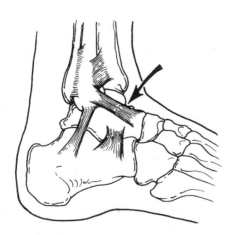
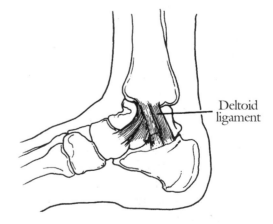

Deltoid ligament

Ankle ligaments.

and the player may feel a tearing sensation, and experience pain. Sometimes, during tackling, if the studs of the boot are fixed in the turf, the ankle can be pushed over, causing disruption to the outside ligament complex. If there is jostling as the player lands after jumping, the player may land unbalanced, and the ankle can easily become twisted.

In the pre-season when the ground is hard, the studs cannot grip and so the amount of boot sole in contact with the turf is less. This is an inherently less stable situation, and can lead to easier inversion.

Another cause is a twisting injury to the whole joint. If studs are fixed, and a rotational force is applied to the rest of the body, the foot can 'twist out' at the ankle causing widespread ligament injury, and often fracture.

In making a diagnosis, the history of this injury is usually clear. The medical team will, after taking the case history, carefully examine the joint. There will usually be some swelling, and there may be some impressive bruising after 12–24 hours. It is important to exclude a fracture, which can occur, and which may look like a severe sprain. Emergency departments often use the 'Ottawa Rules', guidelines which are 100% valid in diagnosing a fractured ankle.

Many players will have X-ray unnecessarily, especially in the professional game, and there are some fears about over-exposure to radiation. MRI scanning, if available, will make things easier to elucidate. When forcing the foot upwards towards the shin, if this is not too painful, if the two ankle bones can be seen to separate a small amount it may mean a much larger extent of injury. Most sprained ankles are not associated with a fracture, but these should not be dismissed as minor injuries. The soft tissues around the ankle, unless

The Ottawa Rules

The ankle is fractured if there is:

- bone tenderness along the lower 6cm of the back part of the outside or inside ankle bones (the tibia and fibula)
- pain when feeling the base of the fifth metatarsal bone
- tenderness when feeling the navicula bone (on the inside of the foot, just in front of the ankle joint itself)
- inability to bear body weight immediately after the injury, or in the emergency room.

treated promptly and properly, can cause long-term problems.

Treatment should be aimed at early mobilization of the joint, and a restoration of normal proprioception. During this phase, to allow normal movement with the very painful ankle, a brace may be used to reduce the insecure feeling that the player may be experiencing.

Proprioception is the body's balance mechanism. It allows the brain to sense when ligaments, tendons and joints are being overstretched, and are moving towards getting injured. When there is an injury to these tissues, the ability to transmit back to the brain is lessened. When this is happening the brain may not be able to co-ordinate correct movement, which makes re-injury more likely. Although this ability is damaged along with everything else in an injury, its function can be recovered just like the other structures. Proprioception can be trained by using a wobble board. Even standing on one leg will help. Once players can do this easily, let them do the same with their eyes closed.

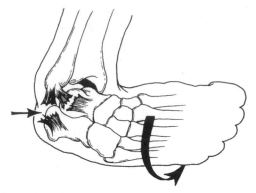

Lateral sprain.

Mobilization is important, as the injured structures will scar and stiffen, delaying recovery. The range of motion of the joint will be limited, increasing the likelihood of re-injury. If the ankle has stiffened, a period of stretching will return it to normal, but this may take time.

Hence, with early physiotherapy aimed at mobilizing the joint, and training back the proprioception that has been lost, the player should be able to play again in 3–4 weeks. If they are unable, a specialist's opinion may be advisable. Occasionally, even with innocuous ankle sprains, the top of the talus bone may get damaged. This can mean that a small piece of the hyaline cartilage covering the bone has become detached. This sometimes happens with a small chip of bone, which can remain tethered, or can float freely around the joint as a loose body. If the ankle does not seem to be rehabilitating to the normal schedule, and becomes more painful or swollen rather than less, this should be suspected. An MRI is the best way to identify this, and surgery is often required though the outcome, especially in adults, is variable.

If the ligaments that join the two ankle bones just above the ankle are disrupted, surgery to bind the two bones together may be necessary, even if there are no fractures (although there often are).

Prevention of ankle sprain is by taping and bracing. There are braces on the market now that can be worn for playing and training. Taping done by experienced practitioners, while not as protective, may be preferred (*see* Chapter 6).

Proprioceptive training has been hailed as the best way to avoid injury, but the hard evidence is difficult to find. There is no doubt that soccer players will have better proprioception than the general population, and the standing, non-dominant side will be better, but whether training this sense will prevent injury is unclear.

Footballer's Ankle

Also called soccer player's ankle, this is a syndrome of ankle damage, rather than injury, associated with soccer. The act of kicking in soccer traumatizes the top of the foot and the lower end of the shinbone with the ball. Occasionally, in a tackle, a player may kick an opponent's boot. As well as the local trauma, the foot is forced backwards during kicking causing a pulling on the structures at the top of the foot.

Both of these set up an inflammatory reaction in the bones involved. When bone becomes repetitively traumatized, it grows extra bits of bone as a protection, and it is the formation of these extra pieces of bone that is called footballer's ankle. The extra pieces of bone are called osteophytes, and can be thought of in the same way as one thinks of calluses on the skin on the hands of manual workers, or of sportspeople, such as windsurfers, who use their hands.

Diagnosis is often made when the syndrome is found incidentally when the ankle has been injured. An X-ray or scan reveals the characteristic extra pieces of bone.

At screening, or profiling, it may be evident that a player can perform a calf stretch equally right and left. The reasons for this are many, but one is that the small outgrowths of bone at the front of the ankle are 'kissing' each other, preventing further stretching of the calf. At this point an X-ray or ultrasound scan will show the presence of the bony outgrowths, and the need to push the player to produce a better stretch can be stopped.

The ankle may not be problematic, and therefore will need no intervention. However, it may become part of the problem in rehabilitation from an ankle or calf injury. If the calf muscles are tight, perhaps tearing recurrently, then stretching them may be impaired by the blockage of movement by a footballer's ankle.

Sometimes the bone growths are so large that they stop the player running properly. During sprinting, the foot has to move up towards the calf (called dorsiflexion). If it cannot, because of a block to the movement, then the player will not be able to run properly. If either of these are the case, then surgical removal is relatively straightforward. Return to play, however, may take 2–3 months.

Os Trigonum Syndrome

About 10% of the population have a small extra piece of bone that extends back from the body of the talus bone of the ankle that swings in between the two main ankle bones. This is called the os trigonum.

Not unlike the extra bits of bone at the front of the joint in footballer's ankle, this bone can get caught between the back of the tibia and the calcaneum (heelbone). It can be felt at the back of the ankle.

A forced flexion of the foot downwards (plantar flexion), as if pointing the toes to the ground, will cause this problem. This can happen during a tackle, where the player is just going to kick the ball, and the opponent misses the ball and makes contact with the foot, forcing it down. The os trigonum is pinched between the two bones.

After asking the player the mechanism of the injury, examination reveals pain when the back of the ankle is felt. Forced plantar flexion, mimicking the injury, brings on the most pain.

X-rays will confirm the presence of an os trigonum, but MRI scanning is the investigation of choice. This may show some damage to the bone and the tendon sheaths that are near it. MRI scanning also allows the medical team to inspect closely the rest of the ankle.

Treatment can be difficult. The normal PRICE regime should be instituted, and non-steroidal anti-inflammatories may be used to reduce inflammation. Strapping may be helpful at this time to avoid accidental movements. If the problem is not settling, steroid injection may be used in an attempt at delivering the anti-inflammatory agent right to the spot where it is needed. It may be useful to do this under ultrasound or fluoroscopic guidance.

If none of these work and recovery has stalled, it may be necessary to resort to surgery, and removal of the offending piece of bone. Recovery takes 2–3 months, and the amount of scarring caused by the operation can delay that recovery.

There is no prevention, except on screening and profiling to note the presence of the os trigonum. At least then, if the player has a minor injury in this area, the correct amount of rest and treatment can be prescribed before it becomes more serious.

THE FOOT

Stress Fracture of the Navicula

The navicula bone sits on the inside of the foot, just in front of the ankle joint. It is at the apex of the arch of the foot. It is in a difficult position, because as the foot collapses during running, it gets pinched between the bones on either side. Also, it is the site for the attachment of one of the main tendons from the muscle that pulls the foot up and inwards, and also one that pulls the foot down and inwards. These opposing forces mean that it comes in for more than its fair share of trauma, sometimes resulting in stress fracture. This injury is more common in those with a high arched foot, which causes greater compressive stress when running, and also is less shock absorbing than the flat foot.

Diagnosis involves taking a case history in which the player reports pain that starts early in a run and gets worse and worse until running is impossible. It is sometimes painful at night, but not stiff in the morning like ligament and tendon problems.

When pressed, the player will experience pain, which can be exquisite. X-rays can be misleading, as the stress fracture often does not show up. An isotope bone scan will show a hot spot, but MRI and spiral CT scan are better at outlining the fracture line and its extent.

There are two ways to treat this: immobilization in a cast or a plastic removable boot

---

Self help for blisters

1   Use a doughnut-shaped pad around the blister to eliminate any more pressure.

2   Use a skin lubricant, such as Vaseline, over the blister to protect from any additional stress.

3   Keep the area clean because the blister may pop on its own and you do not want to invite infection.

---

for six weeks, or surgery with screw fixation. The screw can stay there until the next close-season, and be removed then if necessary. The player must be involved in the decision. The non-surgical method does not always work, so some players will always opt for surgery, especially in the professional game.

Prevention is difficult, because although this problem is more common in those with high arches, it is still prevalent in those with flatter feet. Biomechanical assessment should take account of this risk, so that any symptoms in this area are treated seriously.

Self help to prevent blisters

1   File down any calluses so that blisters do not develop under them.

2   Always wear socks when you are wearing shoes.

3   Use two pairs of socks, especially early in the sport season.

4   Buy shoes with a proper fit and break in new shoes gradually.

Jones Fracture

The Jones fracture is named after a famous Welsh orthopaedic surgeon, Robert Jones. It is a fracture of the fifth metatarsal, and more common in younger players. This bone connects the small toe to the part of the foot between the toes and the ankle. About a centimetre back along the bone, towards the toe itself, the blood supply to this bone is at its lowest. There are two tendons attached in that area pulling on it. It may also be true that in modern boots, with narrower soles at the middle part, this bone protrudes over the edge of the boot, with the sole acting as a fulcrum. When running, these forces combine to cause a stress reaction in the bone at this site. The bone tries to heal, but can fail, and fracture.

In diagnosing this fracture, the history of this injury is very often one where the players will say they had some pain prior to the fracture, but did nothing about it. When examining the foot, there will usually be a fair amount of local swelling, and an X-ray will confirm the fracture.

Treatment falls into two categories, surgical or non-surgical. The non-surgical approach involves immobilization in a cast, and rest. The real problem is that with this approach a large number of players re-fracture the bone. Hence, surgical intervention is the treatment of choice for active sportspeople. This involves placing a screw into the bones that, when tightened, pulls the ends of the bone together. There is still a period of non-weight bearing, and rehabilitation, but in two months the player is usually fit to play. Even with fixation, there is still the possibility of re-fracture. In both situations, this is because of the poor blood supply to this part of the bone.

There is no way to prevent this. There is no proof that new boots make this more common, and research is all but impossible, since any data on the old type of boot and reliable data on injuries are not available.

March Fracture, or Metatarsal Stress Fracture

There are five metatarsal bones, one for each toe. These bones support the toes and act as a connection between the toes and the other bones in the foot. The middle three can sustain stress fractures. These are called march fractures, as they were first described in soldiers, and associated with marching.

Excessive training, or training on hard surfaces, can bring this injury on. It is probably the case that some foot types are unable to adapt easily to harder surfaces, leaving the bones susceptible to the effects of repetitive trauma.

Diagnostically, there is a classic history of stress fracture. The player will usually say that it started gradually, but by the time they tell anyone, the injury has started hurting as soon as they start to run, and gets worse the more they run, until they have to stop.

X-rays usually show thickening of the bone cortex. This is the hard outer part of the bone, and appears as a denser white on the X-ray. If there is any doubt, isotope bone scan will show a hot spot in this area. MRI scanning will show the stress fracture up easily, but MRI is not always readily available.

The treatment is rest. The foot is put into a cast, either permanent or a plastic removable one, and healing takes place in 4–6 weeks. There are some novel treatments for stress fractures. Bone stimulation using electric currents can quicken healing time, and bisphosphonates, a group of drugs used to treat osteoeporosis in the elderly, can also be used.

Treatment often boils down to secondary prevention: prevention often comes to mind only when the player has already had the injury. The best way to prevent this injury is to make sure that individual players are not pushed too hard. It is easy to say that each member of a group all does the same training, but invariably some players do more than others, and care should be taken with this smaller group, and temporization used more astutely.

Toe Fracture

Toe fractures are common, and minor, but can cause great frustration. The cause is always traumatic, either from kicking an opponent, or being trodden on.

When diagnosing this injury, the toe is visibly swollen. The medical team will hear about the traumatic incident, and after examination an X-ray will confirm the diagnosis.

Rest is the only treatment for this. If it is uncomfortable to walk, the player may need a removable plastic brace and can walk in this until normal walking is comfortable. If the player is not in too much pain, play may be possible in 3–4 weeks, but if the toe is still swollen this may be difficult. It must be remembered that players wear boots of a smaller size than their shoes, so any swelling will be more significant than may appear to be the case with the foot out of a boot.

There is no way to prevent this injury, which is a chance traumatic incident.

Subungual Haematoma or Bruised Toenail

When there is bleeding under the toenail it goes dark because the nailbed bleeds. The pressure of the blood causes pain, which can be quite severe.

It is caused by being trodden on by an opponent, or kicking an opponent, accidentally. Boot size is a factor: if the boot is too big, the foot shoots forwards in the boot when the player suddenly stops running and hits the end of the boot, causing bleeding. If the boot is too small, the toe is constantly traumatized, causing bleeding.

Diagnosis is very simple: the toenail goes dark, and the player will complain if the nail is pressed.

Drilling a hole in the nail to release the blood is the only way to alleviate the pain, and this is instantaneous, causing much relief and gratitude on the part of the player. There are battery-operated devices made specifically for this, but a medical (sterile) needle, rotated with controlled pressure can do the same job.

As for prevention, if the cause is a traumatic one, prevention is impossible. If it is because the player has the wrong-sized boots, this can be remedied.

Turf Toe

This is a traumatic injury that occurs to the underside of the 'big toe joint'. In medical terms, this is the first metatarsophalangeal joint, and is the same one that is involved in bunions. Underneath this toe, there is a tendon that runs forward and attaches to the last bone in the big toe. Its action is to point the toe downwards. It is also the tendon that helps pushing off when running. This is protected by two little bones, one on either side of it, called the sesamoids. The joint capsule is also closely associated with these structures.

When the joint is flexed, for instance when standing on tiptoes waiting to spring off, it is at full stretch. If then, someone runs into you, or in some way causes the area to be overstretched, this causes turf toe. The structures underneath that joint become stretched and torn.

Anything that causes overstretching of the structures underneath the toe can cause this: a tackle, being landed on, or landing awkwardly. Very occasionally, the tendon can rupture, and recognizing this can be difficult in the early stages of the injury.

The player may not have a clear idea of the mechanism, but will have a good idea of the area of pain. The underside of the big toe will be painful to touch, and the player will have trouble walking, with the inability to stretch that part of the toe, and this is essential for normal walking. If the tendon is ruptured, the player will not be able to force the toe downwards when resisted.

X-ray will exclude a fracture, although sesamoid fractures are hard to see sometimes, and if one or both of the sesamoids are bi-partite (in two pieces, a normal variation) this can cause confusion. MRI scanning will give a good idea of the soft tissue damage involved.

Treatment begins with the normal PRICE regimen, and non-steroidal anti-inflammatories might help to settle the pain. The recovery depends on the amount of disruption, but because the tendon is so important to normal ambulation, surgery may have to be undertaken.

Prevention is impossible: this is a traumatic injury that is unavoidable.

Plantar Fasciitis

Plantar fasciitis is a common complaint, especially with older athletes. It is an inflammation (-itis) of the connective tissue (fascia) under the foot (plantar). It is said to affect nearly 20% of runners. The soreness is under the foot and in the heel or just forward of the heel. It is usually caused by bruising the tissue on or near the heel. Stepping on a stone is a common cause. Plantar fasciitis may occur in several tissues in the bottom of the foot. The most common area is on or just in front of the heelbone (calcaneus).

The ligaments and tendons that attach to the heel are prone to problems, either from trauma, overstretching, or tightening due to not being stretched often enough. Tight calf muscles and tendons (gastrocnemius and

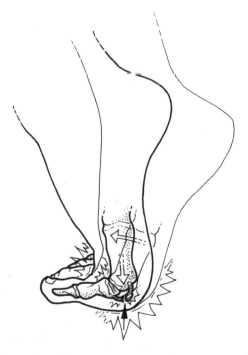

Cause of turf toe.

soleus) are often related to the development of this problem, so stretching of the heel is always recommended as part of the cure. Stretching of the rear calf muscles should be done several times a day.

Another contributing factor is often that the foot is pronated or 'flat': the inside part of the foot is closer to the ground. A proper orthotic device (insole), which lifts the long arch of the foot, may help prevent a recurrence.

The pain is particularly noticeable when getting out of bed in the morning. It may also be evident when arising after being seated for some time. The condition is generally a stress injury where the tendons under the foot are repeatedly stressed, such as in running or in doing heel raises with significant weight on the back.

Relative rest is the most important aspect of treatment. A doughnut pad or a rubber heel cup with extra cushioning underneath may also be an aid. Standard initial treatment should be used, with icing after use of the bruised foot, then doing the hot and cold contrasting baths to increase the healing of the tissue in that area. Relative rest is also a good idea, and a gradual reintroduction of the activity that caused the problem, so the problem is avoided. Using orthotics and/or rubber heel cups will help to reduce the chance of the problem reoccurring. Anti-inflammatory injections often help.

Self help for plantar fasciitis

1. Stretch the Achilles tendon by standing a few feet from a wall, facing it, then allow the hips to drop toward the wall. Bend the ankle forward and feel the pull at the back of the heel.

2. Use a soft rubber heel cup to ease the pain by cushioning the heelbone (and probably the heel spurs) when the heel hits the floor. The heel cup also reduces the tension of the Achilles tendon and the stretch of the ligaments under the foot. You can also use a felt or sponge rubber doughnut with the hole surrounding the spot where it is sore.

3. Use an appropriate orthotic to aid recovery.

4. Wear soft, flexible, well-cushioned shoes, rather than stiff ones.

5. NSAIDs such as aspirin may reduce the inflammation and the pain.

6. Don't walk or run on your toes, walk or run on hard surfaces, or walk in bare feet.

7. Do exercises that strengthen the under-part of the foot. Put a towel on the floor and with your toes over the edge of the towel, bring it towards you by curling the toes under and pulling the towel.

Self help for pump bumps: pain on the back of the heel

1. Use an ice cup in a circular motion to reduce the inflammation.

2. Wear shoes with softer heel sections and which do not put pressure on the Achilles tendon.

3. Use a doughnut pad over the inflamed area.

4. Do not do exercises that use the calf muscle (heel raises, jumping, running).

CHAPTER 23

Special Concerns for Female Players

Women's soccer has grown remarkably. In 1921, the Union of European Football Associations (UEFA) actually banned women's participation in soccer, and the ban was not lifted until 1971. In the USA, women's soccer has probably evolved quicker than anywhere, with 43% of the soccer-playing population being women. In the rest of the world, the figure is 22%.

There is no doubt that there are physical differences between men and women, and there are also differences in the rates of some the injuries inevitably sustained in soccer. Two types of injuries encountered in soccer stand out as being more common in women: knee injuries and stress fractures.

KNEE INJURIES

One research study, done in 1995 in the USA, found that the rate of all knee injuries to women players was 1.6 per thousand exposures, as opposed to 1.3 in men. This is a difference of over 20%. When the anterior cruciate ligament (ACL) rupture rates are examined, the difference is 40%, women greater than men. This is still a serious injury, despite great strides in reconstructive surgery. If the reasons for this are understood then prevention may be at least partly possible.

The reasons why it happens are complex, but need to be examined closely. When the player is running, as the foot hits the floor (heel first), the muscles of the thigh suddenly contract, both hamstrings and quadriceps. Measurements have shown that, at high speeds, the strength to do this with control is less in women. However, the important thing is that, in men, the hamstrings contract first and act to pull on the tibia, stopping it moving forwards. In women it is the quadriceps, and especially the inner part of the quadriceps, that pulls the tibia forwards. This has implications: a proposed mechanism for ACL rupture is that the tibia moves forwards with relation to the femur, and the femur comes up against the top of the tibia, causing the ACL to rupture. Hence, any restraining mechanism will help avoid the injury, but this does not appear to be the case in women. There may be different neuro–muscular patterns at work, and in a sport such as soccer this leaves the player open to this type of injury.

Coupled with this some researchers have found that the biomechanical make-up of some women pre-dispose them to this injury. The angle of the knee when landing from a jump is just one of the variables that has been shown to be of importance.

Apart from the mechanics of the injury, it has been shown that this injury happens more commonly during menstruation ('period'). Some have cited an 'irritability' and 'lack of coordination'. This may be true if there is pain related to menstruation, but again there is no hard research evidence for this. There is some research showing that there are hormonal influences on the regeneration of fibres such as those found during menstruation, perhaps impeding regeneration and adaptation. This is conjecture at present. Certainly women who take the contraceptive pill are less likely than their counterparts to sustain this injury.

With neuro–muscular training, the way the nervous system causes movement and contraction can make a difference. The use of plyometrics, core stability, and greater hamstring strength and co-ordination has been shown to bring down the rate of this injury in women soccer players.

STRESS FRACTURES

Stress fractures in different areas of the body have been dealt with previously in this book. However, stress fractures are more common in women soccer players.

In athletically trained women, menstruation can become irregular, because of a disturbance of the normal way that hormone production is governed by a gland in the brain. Hormones travel to the ovaries, where oestrogen is produced. They are also involved in the process that causes ovulation. One of the things that oestrogen does is to help keep bone strong. Some researchers have shown that women with disturbed periods have less bone density. In those athletes whose periods have stopped altogether (which can occur), and who have a history of stress fracture, the loss in bone density has been measured as up to 49%. Hence, if oestrogen is not at normal levels, the bones will lose some of their density and, with the rigours of soccer training, will be prone to suffering stress fractures. In young athletic women, the start of periods (the menarche) may be delayed.

Most of these studies were done in women athletes where excess weight was a factor (real or perceived) in performance. In women's soccer this is less of a problem than in, say, long distance runners. However, the problem is still present in soccer, albeit much less commonly.

Coupled with the training load causing a disturbance in a woman's periods, some may also manage their food intake to achieve an 'ideal' weight or body type. High intensity training and food management can occur in women soccer players, and if bone density is compromised, this then becomes what has been called the 'female athletic triad'. This is amenorrhoea (no periods at all), osteoporosis (reduced bone density), and the eating disorder anorexia nervosa (or bulimia nervosa).

In the past, it has been stated that the player's weight or body fat content is the determining factor for periods stopping, but there are many women with less body fat than this who still have normal, regular periods. It has more to do with a reduced metabolic rate, linked to high intensity training in the face of a reduced energy intake. Recently, a hormone called leptin has been found, which is produced by fat cells. There is a much closer relationship between the level of this and whether periods are present or not.

A female player whose periods have stopped, even if she is training excessively, and may have an eating disorder, should consult a doctor. The most common cause of periods stopping in young women is pregnancy. There are also other disease processes that can cause periods to cease.

When consulting a doctor, if pregnancy and all the disease processes have been excluded, the doctor may offer the contraceptive pill to the player. This is not for contraception, but for oestrogen replacement. This may lead to some difficult decisions for players, as one of the side effects of the pill is that the woman may put on weight, which is one of the contributory factors to the problem. Reducing training, and increasing food intake will lead to full restoration of the periods, but if a reduction in bone density has been found, the woman should be regularly screened for bone density. Bear in mind that after menopause women's bones may become thinner anyway. This is important if the woman's bone density never recovered when previously lower, as the bones may become dangerously thin.

Glossary

ABDUCTION taking a body part away from the midline of the body, such as raising the arm to the side.

ACUTE a sudden problem.

ADDUCTION bringing a body part back to the body, such as bringing a raised arm back to the side of the body.

AVULSION FRACTURE a break in the bone caused by a ligament or tendon pulling off a bone chip where it is attached.

BURSA a sac of fluid that provides cushioning and protection around a joint.

CARTILAGE a fibrous type of connective tissue. Some cartilage will become bone as the body ages.

COMPRESSION putting pressure on a body part, such as with an elastic bandage.

CONCENTRIC CONTRACTION a muscular contraction during which the muscle is shortening, as when lifting a cup of coffee or lifting a weight over the head.

CONNECTIVE TISSUE a tough tissue that connects bone to bone (ligament), muscle to bone (tendon) or muscle to muscle.

CONTUSION a blow to the soft tissue, such as a muscle, which causes bleeding, and a bruise.

CHRONIC a long-standing problem.

DISC a cartilage-like soft-centred pad that rests between each vertebra and helps to absorb the shock that the back must endure.

DISLOCATION the movement of a bone out of its normal position in a joint.

ECCENTRIC CONTRACTION a muscular contraction during which the muscle is lengthening (stretched) while it is still contracting, as when bending forward from a standing position when the muscles of the back are lengthening (pronounced 'eksentric' not 'eesentric').

EVERSION turning inwards.

EXTENSION opening up the angle of a joint and returning the body part to the straightened position from a flexed position, as when straightening the arm or leg, or bringing the torso upwards from a bent forward position.

FASCIA a sheet or band of connective tissue.

FLEXION bending a part of the body away from the normal standing position, as when bending the torso forward, bringing the hand closer to the shoulder, or bringing the foot closer to the hip by bending at the knee.

FRACTURE a breaking of a bone, caused by a single trauma or by continued stresses (stress fracture). See also Avulsion fracture.

HYPEREXTENSION going past the normal extended position, as when bending backward, or bringing the fingers or toes up past their straightened position.

INVERSION turning inwards.

ISOMETRIC CONTRACTION a muscular contraction in which the joint does not move, as when standing without moving.

LIGAMENT a type of tough connective tissue that holds one bone to another.

MUSCLE an organ that includes contractile tissues that move the joints of the body when it contracts.

NSAIDs non-steroidal anti-inflammatory drugs such as aspirin and ibuprofen.

PLYOMETRICS exercises that use the stretch-shortening cycle, such as repeated bounding jumps.

PRICE acronym for the essentials of treating most injuries: Protection, Rest, Ice, Compression, Elevation.

PRONATION moving a body part to a prone position.

216

PRONE face down, lying on the front, or the hand palm down.

SPASM a sudden and involuntary muscle contraction, such as a cramp.

SPRAIN a stretching of a ligament. It can be mild, as in a simple stretching, or severe, in which the ligament is torn.

STRAIN a stretching injury of a muscle or a tendon that attaches the muscle to a bone.

STRETCH-SHORTENING CYCLE the action within a muscle in which it is stretched then shortened quickly. Jumping off a chair and immediately jumping upwards is such an action, as is striding forward then pushing backward with the leg.

SUBLUXATION a partial dislocation.

SUPINATION moving to a supine position.

SUPINE facing up, lying on the back, or the hand palm up.

TENDON a type of connective tissue that connects muscle to bone.

VERTEBRA one of the bones in the spinal column, protecting the spinal cord.

References

Aagaard P, et al. (1998) 'A new concept for isokinetic hamstring: quadriceps muscle strength ratio', American Journal of Sports Medicine, 26: 231–7.

AAHPERD (2002) Conference of American Alliance for Health, Physical Education, Recreation and Dance, Cincinatti, OH, April 2002. Speakers Duane Knudson, Arnold Nelson, Vinson Sutlive, et al.

Abwender D (1999) Quoted in Christensen D (1999) Science News, Nov 27, 156(22): 348.

Agel J, Arendt EA and Bershadsky B (2005) 'Anterior cruciate ligament injury in national collegiate athletic association basketball and soccer', American Journal of Sports Medicine, Feb, 33(4): 524–9.

Allen LR, Flemming D and Sanders TG (2004) 'Turf toe: ligamentous injury of the first metatarso-phalangeal joint', Military Medicine, Nov, 169(11): xix–xxiv.

Andersen MB and Williams JM (1999) 'Athletic injury, psychosocial factors and perceptual changes during stress', Journal of Sports Science, Sept, 17(9): 735–41.

Andersen TE (2004) 'Video analysis of the mechanisms for ankle injuries in football', American Journal of Sports Medicine, 32:69S–79S.

Andersen TE (2005) 'Video analysis of injury situations and mechanisms in élite football', unpublished doctoral dissertation, Oslo Sports Trauma Research Center.

Andersen TE, Arnason A, Engebretsen L and Bahr R (2004a) 'Mechanisms of head injuries in elite football', British Journal of Sports Medicine, 38: 690–96.

Andersen TE, Engebretsen L and Bahr R (2004b) 'Rule violations as a cause of injuries in male Norwegian professional football: are the referees doing their job?', American Journal of Sports Medicine, 32: 62S–68S.

Arnason A, Sigurdsson SB, Gudmundsson A, Holme I, Engebretsen L and Bahr R (2004) 'Risk factors for injuries in football', American Journal of Sports Medicine, Jan/Feb, 32: 17S–22S.

Arnason A, Engebretsen L and Bahr R (2005) 'No effect of a video-based awareness program on the rate of soccer injuries', American Journal of Sports Medicine, Jan, 33(1): 77–84.

Asami et al. (1976) 'Energy efficiency of ball kicking' in Komi (ed.) Biomechanics, University Park Press, Baltimore, USA.

Askling C, Lund H, Saartok T and Thorstensson A (2002) 'Self-reported hamstring injuries in student-dancers', Scandinavian Journal of Medicine and Science in Sports, Aug, 12(4): 230–5.

Askling C, Karlsson J and Thorstensson A (2003) 'Hamstring injury occurrence in elite soccer players after preseason strength training with eccentric overload', *Scandinavian Journal of Medicine and Science in Sports*, Aug, 13(4): 244–50.

Askling C, Karlsson J and Thorstensson A (2005) 'Hamstring injury occurrence in elite soccer players after preseason strength training with eccentric overload', *Scandinavian Journal of Medicine and Science in Sports*, Feb, 15(1): 65.

Barnett C and Curran V (2003) 'Dementia in footballers', *International Journal of Geriatric Psychiatry*, 18: 88–9.

Bemben MG and Lamont HS (2005) 'Creatine supplementation and exercise performance', *Sports Medicine*, 35(2): 107–25.

Boorman G, *et al.* (1994) 'Toxicology and carcinogenesis studies of ozone', *Toxicology and Pathology*, Sept, 22(5): 545–54.

Broglio SP, Ju Y-Y, Broglio MD and Sell TC (2003) 'The efficacy of soccer headgear', *Journal of Athletics Training*, Sept, 38(3): 220–24.

Broglio SP, Guskiewicz KM, Sell TC and Lephart SM (2004) 'No acute changes in postural control after soccer heading', *British Journal of Sports Medicine*, Oct, 38(5): 561–7.

Cochrane, J, Lloyd D, Besier T and Ackland T (2003) 'Changes in loading on the knee and knee flexion following lower limb training programmes implemented to assess the effect on risk of knee injury and prevention', *Journal of Science and Medicine in Sport*, Dec, 6(4): S89.

Caraffa A, Cerulli G, Projetti M, Aisa G and Rizzo A (1996) 'Prevention of anterior cruciate ligament injuries in soccer. A prospective controlled study of proprioceptive training', *Knee Surgery in Sports Traumatology Arthroscopy*, 4(1): 19–21.

Chomiak J, Junge A, Peterson L and Dvorak J (2000) 'Severe injuries in football players influencing factors', *American Journal of Sports Medicine*, 28: S.

Cordova ML, Cardona CV, Ingersoll CD and Sandrey MA (2000) 'Long-term ankle brace use does not affect peroneus longus muscle latency during sudden inversion in normal subjects', *Journal of Athletic Training*, 35(4): 407–11.

Cornelius WL and Hands MR (1992) 'The effects of a warm-up on acute hip joint flexibility using a modified PNF stretching technique', *Journal of Athletics Training*, Summer, 27(2): 112–14.

Covassin T, Swanik CB and Sachs ML (2003) 'Sex differences and the incidence of concussions among collegiate athletes', *Journal of Athletics Training*, Sept, 38(3): 238–44.

Dadebo B, White J and George KP (2004) 'A survey of flexibility training protocols and hamstring strains in professional football clubs in England', *British Journal of Sports Medicine*, Aug, 38(4): 388–94.

Dauty M, Potiron-Josse M and Rochcongar P (2003) 'Consequences and prediction of muscle lesions in professional football', *Annales de Readaptation et de Medecin Physique*, Nov, 46(9): 601–6.

Delaney JS and Al-Kashmiri A (2004) 'Neck injuries presenting to emergency departments in the United States from 1990 to 1999 for ice hockey, soccer, and American football', *Clinical Journal of Sport Medicine*, Mar, 14(2), 80–87.

Devan M, *et al.* (2004) 'A prospective study of overuse knee injuries among female athletes with muscle imbalances and structural abnormalities', *Journal of Athletics Training*, Sept, 39(3): 263–7.

Diab N and Mourino AP (1997) 'Parental attitudes toward mouthguards', *Pediatric Dentistry*, Nov–Dec, 19(8): 455–60.

Duma S, *et al.* (2005) 'Analysis of real-time head accelerations in collegiate football players', *Clinical Journal of Sports Medicine*, Jan, 15(1): 3–8.

Eaton L (2002) 'Coroner cites football as reason for brain injury', *British Medical Journal*, 325: 1133.

Frische H (1999) 'Growth hormone and body composition in athletes', *Journal of Endocrinological Investigation*, 22(5): 106S–9S.

Fuller CW, Junge A and Dvorak J (2004a) 'An assessment of football referees' decisions in incidents leading to player injuries', *American Journal of Sports Medicine*, Jan–Feb, 32: 17S–22S.

Fuller CW, Smith GL, Junge A and Dvorak J (2004b) 'The influence of tackle parameters on the propensity for injury in international football',

American Journal of Sports Medicine, Jan–Feb, 32: 43S–53S.

Fuller CW, Smith GL, Junge A and Dvorak J (2004c) 'An assessment of player error as an injury causation factor in international football', *American Journal of Sports Medicine*, 32: 28S–35S.

Gisolfi C, Schiller L and Maughan R (1993) *Roundtable on intestinal fluid absorption in exercise and disease*, American College of Sports Medicine.

Giza E, *et al.* (2003) 'Mechanisms of foot and ankle injuries in soccer', *The American Journal of Sports Medicine*, 31: 550–54.

Giza E, Mithöfer K, Farrell L, Zarins B and Gill T (2005) 'Injuries in women's professional soccer', *British Journal of Sports Medicine*, April 1, (39)4: 212–16.

Goga IE and Gongal P (2003) 'Severe soccer injuries in amateurs', *British Journal of Sports Medicine*, 37: 498–501.

Gullick DT (1995) 'Effects of various treatment techniques on the signs and symptoms of delayed onset muscle soreness', PhD thesis from Temple University.

Guo Z, Cupples LA, Kurz A, *et al.* (2000) 'Head injury and the risk of AD in the MIRAGE study', *Neurology*, 54: 1316–23.

Haglund Y and Eriksson E (1993) 'Does amateur boxing lead to chronic brain damage? A review of some recent investigations', *American Journal of Sports Medicine*, 21(1): 97–109.

Hawkins RD, Maltby S, Hulse M, Thomas A and Hodson A (2004) 'The Football Association Medical Research Programme: an audit of injuries in professional football – analysis of hamstring injuries', *British Journal of Sports Medicine*, Feb, 38(6): 36–41.

Heidt RS, *et al.* (2000) 'Avoidance of soccer injuries with preseason conditioning', *American Journal of Sports Medicine*, 28: 659–62.

High D and Howley E (1989) 'The effects of static stretching and warm-up on prevention of delayed onset muscle soreness', *Research Quarterly on Exercise and Sport*, Dec, 60(4): 357–61.

Jacobs SJ and Berson BL (1986) 'Injuries to runners: a study of entrants to a 10,000 meter race', *American Journal of Sports Medicine*, 14(2): 151–5.

Janda DH *et al.* (1995) 'Goal post injuries in soccer', *American Journal of Sports Medicine*, 23(3): 340–4.

Johansson PH, Lindstrom L, Sundelin G and Lindstrom B (1999) 'The effects of pre-exercise stretching on muscular soreness, tenderness and force loss following heavy eccentric exercise', *Scandinavian Journal of Medicine and Science in Sports*, Aug, 9(4): 219–25.

Jolly KA, Messer LB and Manton D (1996) 'Promotion of mouthguards among amateur football players in Victoria', *Australian and New Zealand Journal of Public Health*, Dec, 20(6): 630–39.

Junge A and Dvorak J (2004) 'Soccer injuries: a review on incidence and prevention', *Sports Medicine*, 34(13): 929–38.

Junge A, Dvorak J, Graf-Baumann T and Peterson L (2004a) 'Football injuries during FIFA tournaments and the Olympic Games, 1998–2001: Development and implementation of an injury-reporting system', *American Journal of Sports Medicine*, Jan–Feb, 32(1 Suppl): 80S–89S.

Junge A, Dvorak J and Graf-Baumann T (2004b) 'Football injuries during the World Cup 2002', *American Journal of Sports Medicine*, Jan–Feb, 32(1 Suppl): 23S–27S.

Junge A, *et al.* (2004c) 'Soccer and rugby injuries in youth amateur players: comparison of incidence and type of injury', *Journal of Sport Sciences*, 22, 483: 587.

Junge A, Khouaja F and Dvorak J (2004d) 'Incidence and types of injuries in the Tunisian professional football league', *Journal of Sport Sciences*, 22, 483: 588.

Karlsson J and Andreasson GO (1992) 'The effect of external ankle support in chronic lateral ankle joint instability', *American Journal of Sports Medicine*, 20: 257–61.

Kartal A, Yildiran I, Senkoylu A and Korkusuz F (2004) 'Soccer causes degenerative changes in the cervical spine', *European Spine Journal*, Feb, 13(1): 76–82.

Kerner JA and D'Amico JC (1983) 'A statistical

REFERENCES

analysis of a group of runners', *Journal of the American Podiatry Association*, 73(3): 160–64.

Kirkendall DT, Marchak PM and Garrett WE (2004) 'A prospective 3 year study of the incidence of injury in youth soccer', *Journal of Sport Sciences*, 22, 483: 589.

Knapik JJ, Bauman CL, Jones BH, Harris JM and Vaughan L (1991) 'Preseason strength and flexibility imbalances associated with athletic injuries in female collegiate athletes', *American Journal of Sports Medicine*, Jan–Feb, 19(1): 76–81.

Kohno T, *et al.* (2004) 'Sport injuries of Japanese adolescent soccer players', *Journal of Sport Sciences*, 22, 483: 589.

Koyama Y, Koike A, Yajima T, Kano H, Marumo F and Hiroe M (2000) 'Effects of 'cool-down' during exercise recovery on cardiopulmonary systems in patients with coronary artery disease', *Japanese Circulatory Journal*, Mar, 64(3): 191–6.

Little T and Williams A (2004) 'Effects of differential stretching protocols during warm-ups on high speed motor capacities in professional footballers', *Journal of Sports Science*, 22, 483: 589–90.

Lohmander LS, *et al.* (2004) 'High prevalence of knee osteoarthritis, pain, and functional limitations in female soccer players twelve years after anterior cruciate ligament injury', *Arthritis and Rheumatism*, Oct, 50(10): 3145–52.

Mandengue SH, Atchou G, Etoundi-Ngoa SL and Tsala-Mbala P (1996) 'Effects of preliminary muscular exercise on body temperature, water loss and physical performance', *Sante*, Nov–Dec, 6(6): 393–6.

Matser EJ, Kessels A, Jordan B, Lezak M and Troost J (1998) 'Chronic traumatic brain injury in professional soccer players', *Neurology*, 51: 791–6.

Matser EJ, Kessels AG, Lezak MD, Jordan BD and Troost J (1999) 'Neuropsychological impairment in amateur soccer players', *Journal of the American Medical Association*, Sept 8, 282(10): 971.

Matser EJ, Kessels AG, Lezak MD and Troost J (2001) 'A dose–response relation of headers and concussions with cognitive impairment in professional soccer players', *Journal of Clinical Experimental Neuropsychology*, 23(6): 770–74.

Maughan R and Shirreffs S (2004) 'Exercise in the heat: challenges and opportunities', *Journal of Sports Sciences*, 22: 917–27.

van Mechelen W, Hlobil H, Kemper HC, Voorn WJ and de Jongh HR (1993) 'Prevention of running injuries by warm-up, cool-down, and stretching exercises', *American Journal of Sports Medicine*, Sept–Oct, 21(5): 711–9.

Mjølsnes R, Arnason A, Østhagen T, Raastad T and Bahr R (2004) 'A 10-week randomized trial comparing eccentric vs. concentric hamstring strength training in well-trained soccer players', *Scandinavian Journal of Medicine and Science in Sports*, Oct, 14(5): 311–17.

Naunheim RS, Standeven J, Richter C and Lewis LM (2000) 'Comparison of impact data in hockey, football, and soccer', *Journal of Trauma*, May, 48(5): 938–41.

Naunheim R, *et al.* (2002) 'Does the use of artificial turf contribute to head injuries?', *Journal of Trauma-Injury Infection & Critical Care*, Oct, 53(4): 691–4.

Nieman DC, *et al.* (1997) 'Carbohydrate supplementation affects blood granulocyte and monocyte trafficking but not function after 2.5 hours of running', *American Journal of Clinical Nutrition*, July, 66(1): 153–9.

Nioka S, Moser D, Lech G, Evengelisti M, Verde T, Chance B and Kuno (1998) 'Muscle deoxygenation in aerobic and anaerobic exercise', *Adv Exp Med Biol*, 454: 63–70.

Nosaka K and Clarkson PM (1997) 'Influence of previous concentric exercise on eccentric exercise-induced muscle damage', *Journal of Sports Science*, Oct, 15(5): 477–83.

Nybo L, Secher NH and Nielsen B (2002) 'Inadequate heat release from the human brain during prolonged exercise with hyperthermia', *Journal of Physiology*, Dec 1, 545(2): 697–704.

O'Brien B, Payne W, Gastin P and Burge C (1997) 'A comparison of active and passive warm-ups on energy system contribution and performance in moderate heat', *Australian Journal of Science and Medicine in Sport*, Dec, 29(4): 106–9.

O'Connor B (2001) *Complete Conditioning of the Female Athlete*, Wish Publications.

O'Connor B (2003) 'Stretching: the truth', *Scholastic Coach*, 72(6): 46.

O'Connor B, Budgett R, Wells C and Lewis J (2004) *Prevention and Treatment of Athletic Injuries*, Crowood Press, Wiltshire.

O'Connor, C (1991) 'The relationship among gender, injury severity, and pain beliefs of athletes', Unpublished Master's thesis, Ithaca College, NY.

Olmsted LC, *et al.* (2004) 'Prophylactic ankle taping and bracing: a numbers-needed-to-treat and cost–benefit analysis', *Journal of Athletics Training*, March, 39(1): 95–100.

Olsen OE, *et al.* (2005) 'Exercises to prevent lower limb injuries in youth sports: cluster randomised controlled trial', *British Medical Journal*, Feb, 330: 449.

Piazza O, Siren AL and Ehrenreich H (2004) 'Soccer – neurotrauma and amyotrophic lateral sclerosis – is there a connection?', *Current Medical Research and Opinion*, 20(4): 505–8.

Pickett W, Streight S, Simpson K and Brison RJ (2005) 'Head injuries in youth soccer players presenting to the emergency department', *British Medical Journal*, 394: 226–31.

Pitkanen HT, *et al.* (2003) 'Leucine supplementation does not enhance acute strength or running performance but affects serum amino acid concentration' *Amino Acids*, July, 25(1): 85–94.

Pollard CD, Davis IM and Hamill J (2004) 'Influence of gender on hip and knee mechanics during a randomly cued cutting maneuver', *Clinical Biomechanics*, Dec, 19(10): 1022–31.

Pope RP, Herbert RD, Kirwan JD and Graham BJ (2000) 'A randomized trial of pre-exercise stretching for prevention of lower-limb injury', *Medical Science of Sports and Exercise*, Feb, 32(2): 271–7.

Proske U, Morgan DL, Brockett CL and Percival P (2004) 'Identifying athletes at risk of hamstring strains and how to protect them', *Clinical Experience in Pharmacology and Physiology*, Aug, 31(8): 546–50.

Rahnama N and Manning L (2004) 'The mechanisms and characteristics of injuries in youth soccer', *Journal of Sports Science*, 22, 483: 590–91.

Rarick GL, Bigley G, Karst R and Malina RM

(1962) 'The measurable support of the ankle joint by conventional methods of taping', *Journal of Bone and Joint Surgery*, 44-A: 1183–190.

Rasch PJ and Morehouse LE (1957) 'Effect of static and dynamic exercises on muscular strength and hypertrophy', *Journal of Applied Physiology*, 11: 29–34.

Rodenburg J, *et al.* (1994) 'Warm up, stretching and massage diminish harmful effects of eccentric exercise', *International Journal of Sports Medicine*, Oct, 15(7): 414–19.

Rosenbaum D and Hennig EM (1995) 'The influence of stretching and warm-up exercises on Achilles tendon reflex activity', *Journal of Sports Science*, Dec, 13(6): 481–90.

Scarmeas, *et al.* (2002) 'Premorbid weight, body mass, and varsity athletics in ALS', *Neurology*, Sept, 10(59): 773–5.

Sharpe SR, Knapik J and Jones B (1997) 'Ankle braces effectively reduce recurrence of ankle sprains in female soccer players', *Journal of Athletic Training*, 32(1): 21–4.

Shrier I (1999) 'Stretching before exercise does not reduce the risk of local muscle injury: a critical review of the clinical and basic science literature', *Clinical Journal of Sports Medicine*, Oct, 9(4): 221–7.

Soderman K, Werner S, Pietila T, Engstrom B and Alfredson H (2000) 'Balance board training: prevention of traumatic injuries of the lower extremities in female soccer players? A prospective randomized intervention study', *Knee Surgery Sports Traumatology Arthroscopy*, 8(6): 356–63.

Sortland O and Tysvaer AT (1989) 'Brain damage in former association football players. An evaluation by cerebral computed tomography', *Neuroradiology*, 31: 44–8.

Stalnacke BM, Tegner Y and Sojka P (2004) 'Playing soccer increases serum concentrations of the biochemical markers of brain damage S-100B and neuron-specific enolase in elite players: a pilot study', *Brain Injuries*, Sept, 18(9): 899–909.

Stewart IB and Sleivert GG (1998) 'The effect of warm-up intensity on range of motion and anaerobic performance', *J Orthop Sports Phys Ther*, Feb, 27(2): 154–61.

Terjung RL, Clarkson P, Eichner ER, Greenhaff PL, Hespel PJ, Israel RG, Kraemer WJ, Meyer RA, Spriet LL, Tarnopolsky MA, Wagenmakers AJ and Williams MH (2000) 'American College of Sports Medicine roundtable. The physiological and health effects of oral creatine supplementation', *Medical Science of Sports and Exercise*, Mar, 32(3): 706–17.

Thomassen A, *et al.* (1979) 'Neurological, electroencephalographic and neuropsychological examination of 53 former amateur boxers', *Acta Neurol Scand*, 60(6): 352–62.

Tropp H, Askling C and Gillquist J (1985) 'Prevention of ankle sprains', *American Journal of Sports Medicine*, 13: 259–82.

Vinger PF and Capao FJA (2004) 'The mechanism and prevention of soccer eye injuries', *British Journal of Opthalmology*, 88: 167–8.

Wagenmakers AJ (1999) 'Amino acid supplements to improve athletic performance', *Current Opinion on Clinical Nutrition and Metabolic Care*, Nov, 2(6): 539–44.

Walden M, Hagglund M and Ekstrand J (2005) 'Injuries in Swedish elite football', *Scandinavian Journal of Medical Science in Sport*, 15: 118–25.

Walter SD, *et al.* (1989) 'The Ontario cohort study of running-related injuries', *Archives of Internal Medicine*, 149(11): 2561–4.

Williams MH (1999) 'Facts and fallacies of purported ergogenic amino acid supplements', *Clinical Sports Medicine*, July, 18(3): 633–49.

Witvrouw E, *et al.* (2003) 'Muscle flexibility as a risk factor for developing muscle injuries in male professional soccer players', *American Journal of Sports Medicine*, 31: 41–6.

Index